Present Status of Imaging Modalities For Implant Therapy

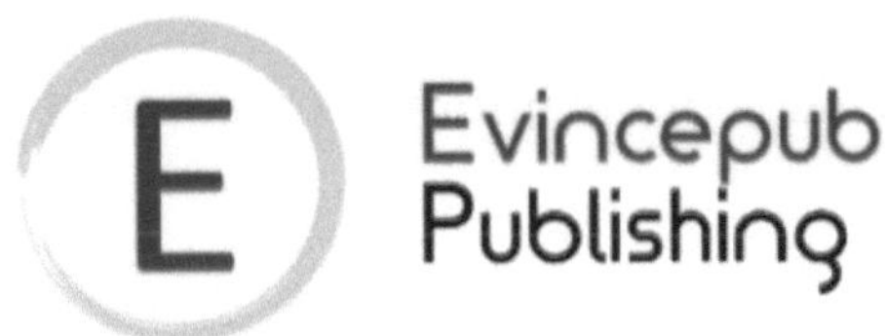

Evincepub Publishing

Nehru Nagar, Bilaspur, Chhattisgarh 495001

First Published by Evincepub Publishing 2021

ISBN: 978-93-5446-198-9

PRESENT STATUS OF IMAGING MODALITIES FOR IMPLANT THERAPY

Dr Jayshri Nandanwar

Dr Manohar Bhongade

Dr Akash Kasatwar

Dr Prasad Dhadse

Acknowledgement

In ancient Japanese culture when an individual set out to accomplish a goal, he or she would hang out a one eyed paper doll at a template's entrance. On fulfillment of this dream, the individual would then place the other eye signifying so and bowing down his head in the acknowledgment.

I am indeed blessed that the goal that I had set out to achieve has taken a step in its fulfillment in the form of this dissertation.

I express my sincere gratitude to my guide **Dr. M. L. Bhongade** for his constant support, supervision, patience and showering of knowledge that I will be benefitted for a long time to come. His valuable suggestions, observations and guidance were the key stone in the making of this dissertation. It has honour to be his student. He has taught and guided me, both consciously and subconsciously. I am also thankful for the excellent example he has provided both as a successful Periodontics and a human being.

This dissertation has taken its shape through the encouragement and insightful comments by my teachers **Dr. Prasad Dhadse** (Professor), **Dr. Vidya Baliga** (Asso. Professor), **Dr. Priyanka Jaiswal** (Asso. Professor), Dr. Kaustubh Thakare, Dr. Preeti Charde, Dr. Pavan Bajaj, Dr. Sneha Puri, Sr. Lecturers in the Dept. of Periodontics & Implantology. I gratefully acknowledge their affectionate motivation, kind suggestions, appraisal and minute analysis that helped me throughout.

I offer with profound respect and immense gratitude my heartfelt thanks to **Dr. R.M. Borle**, Registrar, D.M.I.M.S. university, **Dr. A. J. Pakhan**, Dean, **Dr.Manoj Chandak**, Dean (Academics), Sharad Pawar Dental College and hospital, Sawangi (Meghe), Wardha, for his constant encouragement and support throughout my endeavour during my postgraduation period & also for giving me all the requested co-operation and allowing me to use the facilities of the college during this assignment.

I wish to express my special thanks to my seniors Dr. Kushal, Dr. Noopur, Dr. Roshani, Dr. Ingita, Dr. Prerana and Dr. Komal for their valuable suggestions and ever helping attitude. I am truly lucky to have batchmates Dr. Ashish, Dr. Bushra and Dr. Vikas who have always been on my side through every thick and thin and have been the source of constant encouragement. I sincerely appreciate the help and assistance of my colleagues Dr. Shilpa, Dr. Pooja, Dr. Pranav, Dr. Ankita, Dr. Bhairavi and Dr. Tulika in the Department of Periodontics, their help, support and contribution can't be ignored in successful completion of this task and without whom this could not have been possible.

Someone has rightly said, **"A Father's goodness is higher than the mountain and a Mother's goodness deeper than the sea"**. Nothing of what I have done could be materialized without the unconditional love and cooperation by my parents, **Mr. Arvind &Mrs. Jyoti Nandanwar** their innumerable sacrifices and support during hard and light times of my life have brought me to the position where I stand today. I owe everything to them. Life would have been meaningless without them. I also express my gratitude to my sister, **Mrunalini** and my brother **Ajinkya** for their constant support, love and encouragement that no other source could have provided.

Words will never be enough to express my gratitude for my in-laws **Dr. Pundlikrao & Kumud Kasatwar**, for being a pillar of strength and everlasting support in every endeavour that I partake.

This acknowledgement would be incomplete and unjust without expressing my heartfelt gratitude for my life partner **Dr. Akash Kasatwar**. He has been on my side through all the hard and light times of my life, boosting my morale. His constant encouragement and unwavering faith are a driving force for me in all the spheres of my life. It is due to his persistent support, love, care and understanding that all of this has been possible.

Last but not the least; I thank the God Almighty for giving me courage, wisdom and an opportunity to fulfill my dreams.

I thank God for giving me the strength through all tests in life making my life more plentiful. In God I trust. I will not be afraid. May your name be honoured. Thanks to be God.

Dr. Jayshri A Nandanwar

Authors

1.Dr Jayshri Nandanwar
Consultant Periodontist & Implantologist
Kasatwar's Dental Hospital
Chandrapur-442401
Maharashtra,
India
Email id: jayshrinandanwar@gmail.com

2.Dr Manohar Bhongade,
Consultant Periodontist & Implantologist
Ex Professor & HOD
Sharad Pawar Dental College & Hospital
Datta Meghe Institute of Medical Sciences (DMIMS)
Nagpur,
Maharashtra,
India

3. Dr Akash Kasatwar
Consultant Oral & Maxillofacial Surgeon
Kasatwar's Dental Hospital
Chandrapur-442401
Email id:kasatwaraakash@gmail.com
Maharashtra,
India

4.Dr Prasad Dhadse
Professor & HOD
Sharad Pawar Dental College & Hospital
Datta Meghe Institute of Medical Sciences (DMIMS)
Sawangi (Meghe)
Wardha
Maharashtra
India

Index

CHAPTER 1

INTRODUCTION TO IMAGING FOR IMPLANTS

The use of dental implants in oral rehabilitation has currently been increasing since clinical studies with dental implant treatment have revealed successful outcomes (Turkyilmaz et al, 2008).[1] Successfully providing dental implants to patients, who have lost teeth and frequently the surrounding bone relies on the careful gathering of clinical and radiological information, on interdisciplinary communication and on detailed planning. One of the most important factors in determining implant success is proper treatment planning. The objectives of diagnostic imaging depend on a number of factors, including the amount and type of information required and the period of the treatment rendered. After a decision has been made to obtain images, the imaging modality is used that yields the necessary diagnostic information related to the patient's clinical needs and results in the least radiologic risk (Resnik et al., 2008).[2]

The ideal imaging technique for dental implant care should have several essential characteristics, including the ability to visualize the implant site in the mesiodistal, buccolingual and superioinferior dimensions; the ability to allow reliable, accurate measurements; a capacity to evaluate trabecular bone density and cortical thickness; reasonable access and cost to the patient and minimal radiation risk (Benson and Shetty, 2009).[3] However, there is no ideal imaging technique in the field of oral implantology that would be acceptable for all patients. In dental and medical radiology, a recommended principle when selecting the appropriate radiographic modality is based on radiologic dosage. Obviously, the goal is to choose a radiographic method providing sufficient diagnostic information for treatment planning with the least possible radiation dose and costs for the patient.

Traditionally, conventional radiographic images (two dimensional) e.g., periapical, occlusal, panoramic and cephalometric images have been used to assist practitioners in planning implant treatment. Periapical radiographs are commonly used to evaluate the status of adjacent teeth and remaining alveolar bone in the mesiodistal dimension. In addition they have been used for determining vertical height, architecture and bone quality. Occlusal radiographs are used to determine bucco-lingual dimensions of the mandibular alveolar ridge, but it records only the widest portion of the mandible, which typically is located inferior to the alveolar ridge. In addition, the occlusal view is not useful for the maxillary and because of the anatomical limitations (Benson and Shetty, 2009).[3]Panoramic radiographs is an excellent tool for the overview of the maxillofacial area, including vital structures, such as maxillary sinus, inferior alveolar nerve and nasal fossa. But linear and vertical measurements are unreliable because of foreshortening and elongation of the anatomic structures. Clinicians have been diagnosing, treatment planning, placing and restoring dental implants using periapical and panoramic radiographs to assess bone anatomy for several decades. Two dimensional images have been found to have limitations because of inherent distortion factors and the non-interactive nature of film itself provides. With the advent of technology, Digital Subtraction Radiography (DSR) was introduced to dentistry in 1980s (Bragger U 1988, Webber RL et al 1982).[4,5]

With conventional radiography, a change in mineralization of 30-60% is necessary to be detected by an experimented radiologist (Matteson and Deahl 1996).[6] Also the lesions restricted to cancellous bone could not be detected because of its less mineral contents than cortical bone (Matteson and Deahl 1996)[6] but with

DSR the alveolar bone changes of 1-5% per unit volume and significant differences in crestal bone height of 0.78 mm can be detected (Grondahl and Kullendorff 1988).[7] In addition, defects of at least 0.49mm in depth of cortical bone can be detected whereas a lesion must be at least 3 times larger to be detectable with the conventional radiography techniques (Christgau and Hiller 1998).[8] Furthermore, it can be used to assess the bone at each of three phases of implant treatment, evaluation & maintenance. For a successful DSR, identical contrast and density of the serial radiographs, are essential prerequisites, and long experience shows that this technique is very sensitive to any physical noise occurring between the radiographs and even minor changes leads to large errors in results. Magnetic resonance imaging (MRI) has potential for pre-implant imaging due to the lack of ionizing radiation, but acquisition times can be as long as 30 minutes and there is limited bone information available. MRI is not useful in characterizing bone mineralization or as high-yield technique for identifying bone or dental disease. The reverse is true for CT, as the presence of sclerotic bone in the mandibular body makes the inferior dental canal more obvious.

Diagnostic radiography is essential for implants in pre-operative, intra-operative and post-operative assessment by use of a variety of imaging techniques (Bagchi and Joshi 2012).[9] Since conventional radiographic modalities provide a two-dimensional (3D) representation of three dimensional (3D) structures. Therefore, 3D information is essential for the implantologist before placement of osseointegrated dental implants (Frederiksen 1995).[10] Hence, the advancement of radiographic technology including computed tomography, cone beam CT, DentaScan,Spiral tomography, Linear tomography, Sectional/ Transtomography, Interactive computed tomography, imaging stents and softwares are increasingly considered essential for optimal implant therapy (Tyndall and Brook, 2000).[11] Therefore, the aim of the present review is to examine in depth of the benefits of various radiographic imaging techniques available for implant therapy.

IMAGING MODALITIES FOR IMPLANT PATIENTS:

As a person ages, the accumulation of wear and tear often results in the loss of teeth. Sometimes teeth are knocked out through trauma, but more often they simply fallout through neglect or are extracted because they are no longer viable. This loss of teeth impacts on the patient's everyday life as their speech, appearance and food choices are affected (Jayadevappa 2010, Garg 2007).[12,13]Although removable dentures are an obvious solution, many people opt for the permanence of dental implants. Dental implant technology has undergone dramatic changes in the past few years and has become a significant treatment planning option in restorative dentistry. Long-term success rates are reported to approach 95% or more (Garg 2007).[13]In the past, success has been attributed to increasingly sophisticated imaging technology that has been applied to all phases of implant therapy. Successful implant imaging must recognize that the imaging as well as implant process is prosthetically driven (Garg 2007).[13] Because the ultimate objective of fixture placement is a fundamental esthetic and maintainable restoration, no imaging technique is perfect with each examination carrying some risk of false negative or falsepositive results (Berger 2009).[14] Therefore, the patient's specific needs must be carefully considered. It is indeed a disservice to the patient to use recommended imaging technique based on only consideration of radiation dose, cost or proprietary interest. Several imaging techniques are currently available for presurgical and postsurgical examination (Jayadevappa et al 2010).[12]These may vary from simple two-dimensional views such as panoramic radiographs to more complex views in multiple planes depending on the case and experience of the practitioner.

Selection Of A Radiographic Method:

Selection of radiographic methods should be based on basic principles of radiography like

There should be adequate number and type of images to provide the needed anatomic information, In whatsoever technique used, the patients X-ray beam and imaging receptor should be positioned to minimize distortion, ALARA principle should govern the selection if more than one technique is feasible. The ALARA (As Low As Reasonably Achievable) philosophy recognizes that, no matter how small the radiation dose, some adverse effect may result. Consequently any dose that can be reduced without difficulty, great expense, or inconvenience should be reduced (Garg 2007, Berger 2009).[13,14]

Purpose of Radiography:

The purpose of imaging the implant site is

i. To decide whether the implant treatment is appropriate for the patient.

ii. To know the location of vital anatomical structure (inferior alveolar nerve, extention of maxillary sinus).

iii. For the assessment of quantity of bone, height of alveolar process, buccolingual width and angulation,

iv. To identify any possible pathological conditions.

v. To estimate the number, length and width of the implant.

vi. Possible need for additional treatment for instance bone augmentation procedure and to estimate the prognosis.

Imaging Objectives:

The decision of when to image along with which imaging modality to use depends on the three phases:

1. Preprosthetic implant imaging (Phase1): The objectives of this phase are to determine the quantity, quality, and angulation of bone; the relationship of critical structures to the prospective implant sites; and the presence or absence of disease at the proposed surgery sites.
2. Surgical and Interventional implant imaging (Phase2): The objectives of this phase are to evaluate the surgery sites during and immediately after surgery, assist in the optimal position and orientation of dental implants, evaluate the healing and integration phase of implant surgery, and ensure abutment position and prosthesis fabrication are correct.
3. Post prosthetic implant imaging (Phase 3): It commences just after the prosthesis placement and continues as long as implant remains in the jaws. The objectives of this phase are to evaluate the long-term maintenance of implant rigid fixation and function, including the crestal bone levels around each implant, and to evaluate the implant complex.

IMAGING MODALITIES:

There are many imaging modalities that have been employed for implant imaging, including devices developed specifically for dental implant imaging. These modalities can be described as either analog or digital and two dimensional or three-dimensional (Garg et al 2007).[12] Analog imaging modalities are the periapical, occlusal, panoramic, lateral, cephalometric radiographs which are two dimensional systems that employ X-rayfilm and/or intensifying screens as the image receptors (Berger et al 2009).[14] These imaging modalities include conventional radiography like periapical, panaromic, occlusal and cephalometric, substraction radiography, MRI, computed tomography, cone-beam CT, Denta Scan, linear, spiral, sectional, interactive tomography and various imaging softwares along with imaging stents used while implant placement. These create a three-dimensional image which is described not only by its width, height and pixels, but additionally by its depth and thickness.

CHAPTER 2

CONVENTIONAL RADIOGRAPHY

The goal of modern dentistry is to restore the patient to normal contour, function, comfort, esthetics, speech and health, whether by removing caries from a tooth or replacing several teeth. What makes implant dentistry unique is the improved ability to achieve this goal, regardless of the atrophy, disease or injury of the stomatognathic system (Miles DA 2008).[15] However, the more teeth a patient is missing, the more challenging this task may become. As a result of continued research, diagnostic tools, treatment planning, implant designs, materials and techniques, predictable success is now a reality for the rehabilitation of many challenging clinical situations (Misch CE. 1990, Sonick et al 1994).[16,17] Dental implantology has experienced explosive growth during last few years. Treatment planning for implants includes a radiographic examination that provides information about the location of anatomical structures, the quality and quantity of available bone, the presence of infrabony lesions, the occlusal pattern and the number and size of implants as well as prosthesis design, all which are essential for successful implant treatment (Adell R 1981, Engelman et al 1988).[18,19]

The imaging objectives are to provide the clinician with cross-sectional views of the dental arch for visualization of spatial relationship of internal structures of the maxilla and mandible. Minimal image distortion permits accurate measurement. Ideally, the images should allow evaluation of the density of trabecular bone and thickness of the cortical plates bone quality. Imaging studies should help to determine the optimum position of implant placement relative to occlusal loads. In addition, detection of the presence or absence of pathoses and which is assessable at a reasonable cost to the patient are the desirable features (Monsour and Dudhia 2008).[20] The decision of when to prescribe imaging depends upon the integration of these factors and can be organized into three phases. Those are: (1) Pre-surgical implant imaging, (2) surgical and interventional implant imaging. (3) post prosthetic implant imaging. Although several image diagnostic methods are available to evaluate proposed sites for implants, currently, not a single technique is considered ideal for pre- and post-operative analyses. Therefore, few authors suggest a combination of various techniques to obtain reliable information (Frederiksen NL 1995, Silverstein et al 1994).[10,21] However, when weighing risk and cost against the benefit, excessive utilization of newer techniques should be avoided, especially when conventional methods are similarly efficient and adequate.

A. INTRAORAL RADIOGRAPHY:

Intraoral periapical and occlusal radiography images of perhaps the greatest details of any imaging techniques. The paralleling technique with positioning instruments should be used to enable a reliable projection of the anatomic structures on plain views. Good quality intraoral radiographs help to reveal minute pathologic changes of the periodontium and the teeth, which can interfere with implant placement. Attaching film holders to the tube, while carefully positioning the jawbone under investigation parallel to the film, may offer a solution. Alternatively, a positioning device connected to the implants has been proposed to guarantee parallelism between film and implant (Meijer et al 1992).[22] They are used in initial phase of patient evaluation to detect the presence of pathosis, the approximate location of anatomic structures such as maxillary sinus and also estimate the quality of the trabecular bone (Garg et al 2007).[13] When periapical radiographs are used, it is important to ascertain certain guidelines. It is paramount that exposure be made using paralleling angle technique. However, because the film plane can rarely be placed parallel particularly in edentulous areas, the target film distance is difficult to standardize (Berger 2009).[14] Hence, periapical radiographs do not provide an accurate assessment of vertical bone dimension or precise position of critical anatomic structures. As periapical radiographs are unable to provide a cross sectional information, occlusal radiographs are sometimes used to determine the faciolingual dimensions of the mandibular alveolar ridge. Although somewhat useful, the occlusal image records only the widest portion of the mandible which is located inferior to the alveolar ridge. This may give the clinician a wrong impression that more bone is available in the cross-sectional dimension than that actually exists. The occlusal technique is not useful in maxillary arch because of anatomic limitations.

a. Periapical Radiography:

Traditionally, conventional radiographic images e.g., periapical and panoramic images have been used to assist practitioners in planning implant treatment. Periapical radiographs commonly are used to evaluate the status of adjacent teeth and remaining alveolar bone in the mesiodistal dimension. In addition they have been used for determining vertical height, architecture and bone quality (bone density, amount of cortical bone and amount of trabecular bone). Although readily available and relatively inexpensive, periapical radiography has geometric and anatomic limitations. If the paralleling technique is not used, periapical radiographs create an image with foreshortening and elongation (Benson & Shetty, 2009; Chan et al., 2010).[3,23] When the x-ray beam is perpendicular to the film, but the object is not parallel to the film, foreshortening will occur. If the x-ray beam is oriented perpendicular to the object but not the film, elongation will occur. The most accurate intraoral radiographic technique used for implant planning is the paralleling technique. The long cone paralleling technique for exposing periapical radiographs is the technique of choice for the following reasons: Reduced skin dose; minimal magnification; a minimally distorted relationship between the bone height and adjacent teeth is demonstrated; and minimal superimposition of the zygomatic process of the maxilla over the upper molar region. It should be remembered that to get the most from the long cone paralleling technique, it should be performed using a long collimator with a film-focal distance of approximately 30 cm. (Tyndall et al 2000).11 Therefore, standardized periapical radiographs with bite-blocks by using paralling technique should be perform to the longitudinal studies (Benson & Shetty, 2009; Resnik et al., 2008).3,2

Formoso et al (2011)24 analysed the precision of the modification of the long cone parallel technique that can be used with important anatomical limitations & checked the influence of the reference points definition of objects to be measured by using both the original and the modified radiographic techniques. A total of 28 Straumann implants of bone level type were used measuring 4.1 mm in diameter with lengths of between 10 mm and 12 mm. 2 intraoral radiographs were taken of 28 implants with 2 different methods: a standard paralleling technique and a modified technique that used a smaller film and a silicone spacer to ensure parallelism. Measurements of peri-implant bone levels and implant width were made in triplicate on digitized film radiographs. The results of the peri-implant bone levels were that with the parallel method the mean was 0.44 mm and the precision was 0.43 mm, and with the modified method the mean was 0.73 mm and the precision was 0.66 mm. In addition to the correct localization of the point of reference in this study, the precision with the parallel method was 0.08 mm and with the modified method was 0.13 mm. Authors concluded that although it was greater with the gold standard technique than with the modified technique, precision was very high for both methods and accurate enough for clinical use.

Hansen et al (2003)25 compared the DNB technique with conventional intraoral radiography in the assessment of marginal bone loss around dental implants in the mandible and to evaluate observer agreement. Forty patients were included in this study for the follow up examination after treatment with branemark dental implants in lower jaw. Implants were randomly selected if same patient had more than one implant in the same region. Ten implants were selected from each of four dental regions (molars, incisors, canine, premolar) and no more than one implant was selected from same patient. Seven observers assessed all the radiographs and asked to assess the marginal bone level by counting the number of threads between implant- abutment connection and the level of marginal bone on the mesial and distal surfaces of the implant. Three of the observers made all the assessment twice and resulted that the seven observers agreed on the marginal bone level at only 12 of the 80 implant surfaces of these 12 cases, 10 were periapical, 2 were DNB radiographs. In these 12 cases, marginal bone level was assessed superior to thread 1. Inter observer agreement, expressed as the kappa value for 7 observer, was 0.33 for periapical radiograph &0.27 for DNB radiography. The kappa value for the observer assessment of value 0 was 0.5 all other kappa values for the several observers assessments at specific level were < 0.5. The rated kappa value for intra-observer agreement range from 0.75-0.99 for DNB radiography and from 0.94-0.98 for periapical radiography. Author concluded that Scanora multimodal radiography simplifies examination of implant in mandible & observers vitiations is comparable with that of IOPA.

Anil et al (2007)26 described the use of radiographic imaging software to calibrate and measure anatomical landmarks to overcome inherent distortions associated with dental radiographs.

Diagnostic imaging is an essential component of implant treatment planning, and a variety of advanced imaging modalities have been recommended to assist the dentist in assessing potential sites for implants. Although technological advances have resulted in new imaging innovations for implant dentistry, dental radiography remains the most widely used tool for determining the quantity and quality of alveolar bone as it is a non-invasive procedure. However, the unreliable magnification factor associated with conventional radiographs remains a major problem when estimating the amount of bone available at the implant site. Authors concluded that the application of digital technology as well as the improvements in conventional radiographic techniques has facilitated the quality of radiographs and reduced the distortion in panoramic radiography.

In the pre-prosthetic phase, these films are most often used for single tooth implants in regions of abundant bone width. These are well suited for documentation and assessment of possible peri-implant bone resorption during follow-up. However, It is of limited value in determining quantity since the image is magnified, may be distorted, and does not depict the third dimension of bone width. It does not help to determine bone density or mineralization (Kircoset al 2005).2

Fig. 1

Periapical Radiographs Showing Implants in Position

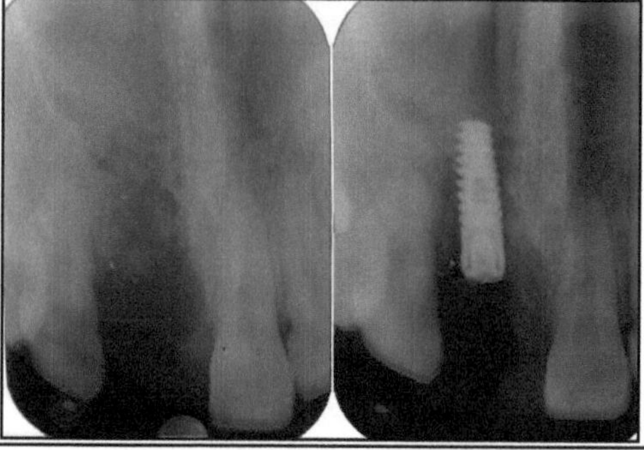

Pre-Operative and Post-Operative Assessment of Implant Sites

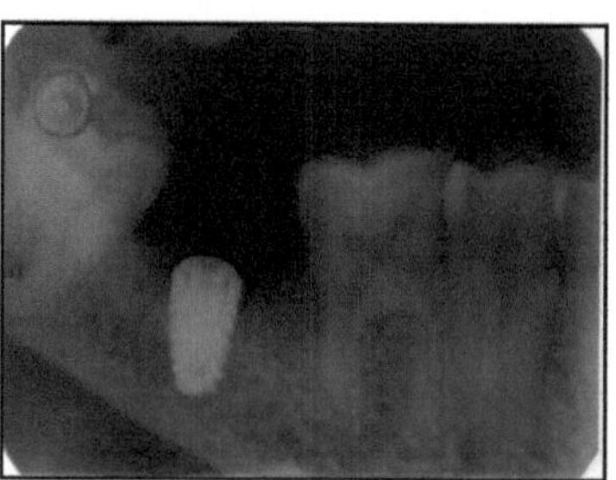

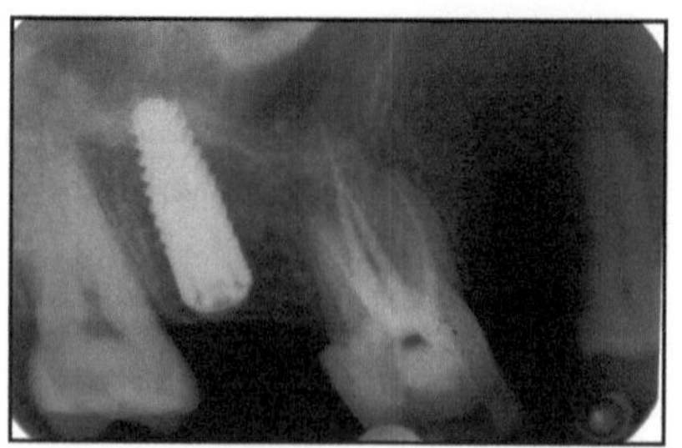

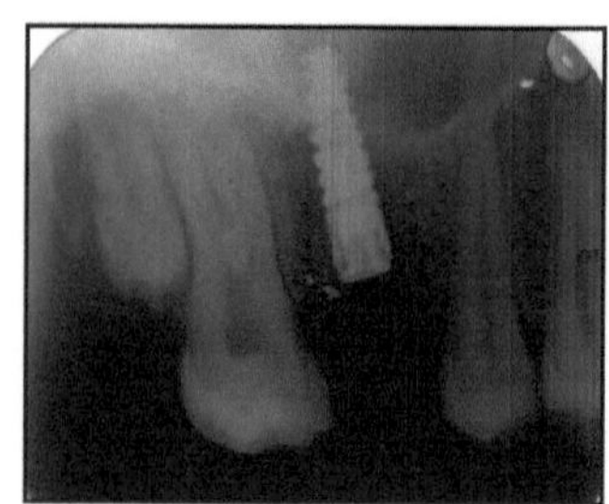

Post-Operative Assessment of Single Tooth Implant in Position

b. Occlusal Radiography :

Occlusal radiographs are planar radiographs produced by placing the film intra orally parallel to the occlusal plane with the central x-ray perpendicular to the film for the mandibular image and oblique (45°) to the film for maxillary image. periapical radiographs are unable to produce any cross sectional information occlusal radiographs are sometimes used to determine the bucco lingual dimensions of the mandibular alveolar ridge Cross-sectional occlusal radiographs of the mandible give some information about the buccolingual dimension of the mandible, but this information is only accurate with regard to the inferior aspect of the body and not the width of the alveolar ridge where the implant is to be placed. The use of cross-sectional occlusal radiographs can be helpful when assessing the position of the implant within the jaw following placement both in the mandible and maxilla.

Jameel et al (2014)[28] evaluated the accuracy of longitudinal topographic occlusal view (LTO) in the measurement of alveolar bone thickness, and designing the beam aiming device to improve technical application of radiographic technique. the alveolar bone thickness of 20 posterior edentulous sites (10 sites for each jaw) in the maxilla and mandible of three dry skulls measured directly by using digital caliper and radiographically by longitudinal topographic occlusal view with newly designed beam aiming device. Statistical analysis of the results with independent paired t-test showed no significant difference between the direct and radiographic bone thickness ($p \geq 0.05$). Authors concluded that the longitudinal topographic occlusal radiograph presents accurate measurements of alveolar bone thickness in the simple and uncomplicated implant cases of the proposed posterior implant sites to avoid the excessive radiation dose, cost and for time saving for patient and operator. The designed beam aiming device recommended using for standardization, and simplicity of technical application.

Maxillary occlusal radiographs are inherently oblique and are so distorted that they are of little quantitative use for implant dentistry, for either determining the geometry or the degree of mineralization of the implant site. In addition, it shows the widest width of bone (i.e. the symphysis) versus the width at the crest, which is where diagnostic information is needed most (Kircos et al 2005).[27]

B. PANORAMIC RADIOGRAPHY:

Assessment of available alveolar bone and bone morphology, with clinical examination and palpation of the bone ridge at the implant site, is essential in preoperative implant planning. Various presurgical imaging techniques, including conventional radiographs (intraoral and panoramic radiographs, occlusal, cephalometry) and computed tomography (CT), are proposed .But there are some limitations of intraoral and occlusal radiography like the periapical radiographs are unable to provide any cross-sectional information and cross sectional occlusal radiographs of mandible give some information about the buccolingual dimension of the mandible, but this information is only accurate with regard to the inferior aspect of the body, not the width of the alveolar ridge where the implant is to be placed. Panoramic radiographs are commonly used for diagnostic purposes in implantology (Dula et al. 2001).29 Three types of shadows can be identified on pantomographs. Structures inside and outside the trough, whose long axis is parallel to the direction of the beam (i.e, structures near the midsagittal plane), form distinct images called primary shadows. Dense structures outside the focal trough, whose long axis is perpendicular to the direction of beam movement, form indistinct images called secondary shadows. Their appearance results from the beam passing the right and left jaw arches simultaneously, so that the jaw side nearest the film forms the primary shadows, while the jaw side nearest the x-ray source produces secondary shadows. The secondary shadows are reversed when the structures near the x-ray source are located behind the center of the beam rotation. Superimposition of secondary and primary shadows can produce apparent radiolucencies caused by contrast. These images are called false shadows because they lack anatomic basis. Although the need for cross-sectional imaging has been strongly recommended (Lindh et al. 1995; Bolin et al. 1996; Bou Serhal et al. 2000; Tyndall & Brooks 2000; White et al. 2001),30,31,32,11,33 panoramic radiography is considered to be the standard radiographic examination for implant treatment planning as it imparts a low radiation dose.

Dharmar et al (1997)34 determined whether it is possible to locate the anteroposterior course of the mandibular canal and the mental foramen more clearly on panoramic radiographs by tilting the patient's head downward approximately 5 degrees with reference to the Frankfort horizontal plane (FHP) of the Orthopantomogram (OPG) machine. One panoramic view would be taken with the standard setting as prescribed by the manufacturer, ie, the FHP of the patient's FHP would be kept at a 5-degree angle downward to the reference bar of the machine. 175 radiographs taken in position 1, a total of 66 were from males (mean age 19.7 years) and 109 were from females (mean age 18.7 years). Twenty-one of these records belonged to a mixed dentition group. All radiographs were taken within a period of 6 months. Position 2 radiographs were taken by positioning the patient's head 5 degrees downward relative to the FH reference plane of the OPG machine. These radiographs were taken over a period of 3 months, as the Departments of Orthodontia and Oral Surgery made requests for diagnostic purposes. Of the 75 radiographs taken with position 2, 40 were from males (mean age 18.6 years) and 35 were from females (mean age 16.4 years). Seventeen records belonged to patients with a mixed dentition. All radiographs were taken by the same radiographer and were developed in the manner prescribed by the manufacturer. The radiographs were read by the author for location of the mental foramen, mandibular foramen, and the entire course of the mandibular canal on both right and left sides. In 91% of the radiographs taken in this position, the mandibular foramen, mandibular canal, and mental foramen were visible. The angulation of the patient's head reduced the chances of superimposition on the contralateral sides, making these structures clearly visible. Authors concluded that by tilting the patient's head 5 degrees downward with reference to the Frankfort horizontal bar of the OPG machine, the mandibular canal can possibly be made more visible.

Vazquez et al(2011)35 estimate a panoramic unit's vertical magnification factor (MF) by measuring the length of dental implants used as radiopaque reference objects on postoperative panoramic radiographs. Using a digital calliper, they measured the length of 32 implants on 17 postoperative panoramic radiographs taken with a Scanoras unit. The implants were 10mm-long placed in the posterior segments of mandibles. The MF was calculated by dividing the implant's radiological length by the implant's real length. The mean calculated vertical MF was 1.27 (1.245–1.295) and was lower than the manufacturer's MF (1.3). The vertical MF was 1.28 in the premolar and 1.27 in the molar regions. There was an excellent intraobserver reliability (0.96 for observer 1; 0.93 for observer 2) and a good interobserver reliability (0.85 at measurement session 1; 0.8 at measurement session 2). Author concluded that reliability of the MF confirms that a panoramic radiograph can be used for preoperative implant length evaluation in the posterior mandibular segments. MF stability should be verified with other panoramic units. In clinical practice, using the implant length as a reference object on postoperative panoramic radiographs is a simple and effective evaluation method to estimate a panoramic unit's MF. Naujem et al (2011) compared the image geneated by classic panoramic machine equipped with a cadmium telluride sensor capable of digital tomosynthesis & special software with images produced by other popular panoramic X-ray machines using a charge -coupled device & native software for image capture. A standardized answer sheet was provided to the viewers, they were instructed to examine the specific ROI (Region of Interest) on the images from each 5 modalities ANOVA for repeated measures was used to compare the means by pairwise comparison of means & resulted that the means over the 10 rates for machines & location varies from 1.0 to 4.7. Five modalities were significantly different overall within raring modalities 2.82, 2.55, 2.40, 2.32, 3.75 respectively. Modalities 2 & 3 were not significantly different in mean rating overall. Modalities 3 & 1 were different ($P < 0.01$) with modality 1 better. Modality 4 was significantly different from all other modalities in overall mean score ($P < 0.007$), as was modality 5 ($P < 0.007$). Modality 5 was statistically superior to l other modalities. The images generated & individually adjusted by PanoACT were statistically superior to all other images. Authors concluded that images generated by the cadmium telluride sensor has great potential & can be processed to create superior image to those taken with other machine. Furthermore, the ROI individual images enhanced by the PanoACT were superior to the entire arch adjusted by the same software.

Gijbels et al (2005)37 compared patient radiation doses generated by five different types of digital panoramic units. An anthropomorphic phantom was filled with thermoluminescent dosemeters (TLD 100w) and exposed with five different digital panoramic units during ten consecutive exposures. Four machines were equipped with a direct digital CCD (charge coupled device) system, whereas one of the units used storage phosphophosphor plates (indirect digital technique). The exposure settings recommended by the different manufacturers for the particular image and patient size were used: tube potential settings ranged between 64 kV and 74 kV, exposure times between 8.2 s and 19.0 s, at fuse current values between 4 mA and 7 Ma & resulted that effective radiation doses ranged between 4.7 mSv and 14.9 mSv for one exposure. Salivary glands absorbed the most radiation for all panoramic units. When indirect and direct digital panoramic systems were compared, the effective dose of the indirect digital unit (8.1 mSv) could be found within the range of the effective doses for the direct digital units (4.7–14.9 mSv). Authors concluded that various digital panoramic machines can provide a rather broad range of effective radiation doses for the patient (4.7–14.9 mSv).

Kim et al (2011)37 evaluated the efficacy and accuracy of cases in which pre-implant diagnosis as well as treatment protocols were prepared through the application of the digital panoramic radiation system without performing CT and other expensive precision tests. He selected 221implants (124 in males, 97 in females) were consecutively placed at the dental clinic in the Seoul National University Bundang Hospital. All of the patients enrolled in this study were partially edentulous or had single missing teeth. On all patients, digital panoramic radiographs were taken before the treatment and after implant surgery. For 10 of the 86 patients, CT was also performed before surgery (4 males, 6 females). They analysed the magnification rate and the difference between the actual inserted implant length and planned implant length according to the location of the implant placement and the clarity of anatomical structures seen in the panoramic radiographs .There was no significant difference between the planned implant length and actual inserted implant length (P. 0.05). The magnification rate of the width and length of the inserted implants, seen in the digital panoramic radiographs, was 127.28¡13.47% and 128.22¡4.17%, respectively. The magnification rate of the implant width was largest in the mandibular anterior part and there was a significant difference in the magnification rate of the length of implants between the maxilla and the mandible (P, 0.05). When the clarity of anatomical structures seen in the panoramic radiographs is low, the magnification rate of the width of the inserted implants is significantly higher (P, 0.05), but there is no significant difference between the planned implant length and actual inserted implant length according to the clarity of anatomical structures (P, 0.05).Authors concluded that the digital panoramic radiography system is an effective method that is simple and inexpensive for pre-implant diagnosis and establishing treatment protocol, and it uses a relatively low radiation exposure.

Vazquez et al (2013)38 assessed the accuracy of the vertical height measurement on post-operative digital panoramic radiographs using implants in the posterior segment of the mandible as intrabony radio-opaque objects. Direct digital panoramic radiographs, performed using a Kodak 8000C of 17 partially edentulous patients (10 females, 7 males, mean age 65 years) were selected from an X-ray database gathered during routine clinical evaluation of implant sites. 9 (36%) implants were inserted in the premolar region and 16 (64%) in the molar region. 15 implants (60%) were located in the left posterior segment of the mandible and 10 on the right side. 11 subjects had a single implant, 5 had 2 implants and 1 had 4 implants. Proprietary software and a mouse-driven calliper were used to measure the radiological length of 25 implants and 18 metal reference balls, positioned in mandibular posterior segments. The distortion ratio (DR) was calculated by dividing the radiological implant length by the implant's real length and the radiological ball height by the ball's real height. Mean vertical DR was 0.99 for implants and 0.97 for balls, and was unrelated to mandibular sites, side, age, gender or observer. Inter- and intraobserver agreements were acceptable for both reference objects. Authors concluded that Vertical measurements had acceptable accuracy and reproducibility when a software-based calibrated measurement tool was used, confirming that digital panoramic radiography can be reliably utilized to determine the pre-operative implant length in premolar and molar mandibular segments.

Fortin et al (2011)39 compared clinically & radiographically panoramic images versus three-dimensional planning software for oral implant planning in atrophied posterior maxillary. During a 2-year period, every patients who presented for the placement of implants in the posterior maxilla were included in this study. Primary planning was based on an intraoral or a panoramic radiograph. When indicated a sinus lift with creation of a lateral window, a CT scan was performed and examined using dedicated three-dimensional software by a clinician familiar with the Computer Assisted Design/ Computer Assisted Manufacturing (CAD/CAM) implant placement protocol. A conventional radiographic guide made of transparent acrylic resin and radiopaque teeth were made. Axial images via multislice CT were then made with the radiographic guide in the mouth. The time between the two radiographic examinations varied from 1 to 3 months. CT images were then examined using the three dimensional Easy-Guide® planning software. For each tooth to be replaced, the presence of anatomical features such as anterior or posterior wall, palatal curvature, and septa were examined in view of the placement of an 8-mm or longer implant. One hundred one patients were studied for the treatment of 135 edentulous spans accounting for 301 missing teeth. After examination of the CT data on the three-dimensional software, 202 teeth (67.1%) could be replaced using a CAD/CAM procedure; 60.7% of the edentulous spans could be completely repaired by a crown or bridge supported by implants. In addition, 67.3% of edentulism with no teeth posterior to the span could be completely repaired using a fixed prosthesis supported by implants. Authors concluded that the use of a panoramic radiological exam for oral implant planning in severely resorbed maxillae overestimates the need for a sinus augmentation procedure, when compared with the use of both three-dimensional planning software and strategic implant placement when there is little remaining bone volume.

Penarrocha et al (2004)40 compared extraoral panoramic with conventional and digital intraoral periapical radiography to quantify marginal bone loss. A total of 108 implants were placed (59 in the maxilla and 49 in the mandible) in 42 patients (16 men and 26 women) with a mean age of 44.2 years (range 14 to 68 years). Orthopantomographic, conventional periapical, and digital radiographs were obtained at loading and again 1 year later. Bone loss was calculated from the difference between the initial and final measurements. Mean loss in alveolar bone height was determined to be 1.36 mm by extraoral panoramic radiography, 0.76 mm by intraoral periapical radiography, and 0.95 mm by digital radiography. The implants located in the maxilla and those placed in patients who smoked 11 to 20 cigarettes per day were associated with significantly greater bone loss. Authors concluded conventional periapical films and digital radiographs were more accurate than orthopantomography in the assessment of peri-implant bone loss. Smoking and implant location in the maxilla were associated with increased peri-implant marginal bone resorption.

Takeshita et al (2014)41compared diagnostic accuracy between conventional, digital periapical radiography, panoramic radiography and cone-beam computed tomography in the assessment of alveolar bone loss. The sample consisted of 70 teeth from 10 macerated human mandibles of the university's Department of Morphophysiology Sciences, each mandible with varied number of teeth. The control method of measuring alveolar bone loss (ABL) consisted of determining the linear distance between the CEJ and the alveolar bone crest on the interproximal surface of the teeth (the CEJ-ABC distance), with the use of a digital calliper accurate to 0.01 mm directly on the mandibles (control), using conventional periapical radiography with film holders (Rinn XCP and Han-Shin), digital periapical radiography with complementary met al-oxide semiconductor sensor, conventional panoramic, and cone-beam computed tomography (CBCT). Three programs were used to measure ABL on the images: Image tool 3.0 (University of Texas Health Sciences Center, San Antonio, Texas, USA), Kodak Imaging 6.1 (Kodak Dental Imaging 6.1, Carestream Health®, Rochester, NY, USA), and i-CAT vision 1.6.20. Statistical analysis used ANOVA and Tukey's test at 5% significance level. The tomographic images showed the highest means, whereas the lowest were found for periapical with Han-Shin. Controls differed from periapical with Han-Shin ($P < 0.0001$). CBCT differed from panoramic ($P = 0.0130$), periapical with Rinn XCP ($P = 0.0066$), periapical with Han-Shin ($P < 0.0001$), and digital periapical ($P = 0.0027$). Conventional periapicals with film holders differed from each other ($P = 0.0007$). Digital periapical differed from conventional periapical with Han-Shin ($P = 0.0004$).Authors concluded that conventional periapical with Han-Shin film holder was the only method that differed from the controls. CBCT had the closest means to the controls.

These are narrow beam rotational tomographs, which use two or more centers of rotation to produce an image, with a predefined focal trough, of both the upper and lower jaws. Panoramic radiography allows complete visualization of the relationship of the maxillofacial structures within the focal trough, and provides information on the relative position of the inferior alveolar canal and the maxillary sinuses in relation to the crest of the alveolar ridge. It provides an approximation of bone height and vital structures and any pathological conditions that may be present (Strid et al 1985).42 A panoramic image cannot provide clinicians with information about the buccolingual cross-sectional dimension or the inclination of the alveolar ridge (Fredholmet et al 1993).43 Angular measurements taken from panoramic radiographs tend to be accurate, but this is not true for linear measurement (Shetty and Benson 1999).44 Assessments of mesiodistal distance can be very imprecise due to inappropriate patient positioning and/or individual variations in jaw curvature (Langland et al 1989).45 The focal trough of panoramic radiography is relatively thick, approximately 20 mm in the posterior region and 6 mm in the anterior region . Moreover, the maxillary and mandibular anterior regions often appear blurred. Due to the use of an intensifying screen to reduce the radiation dosage, panoramic radiographs provide inferior images. Although panoramic radiographs may provide a useful overview and may be used in conjunction with ridge mapping or other diagnostic tools, they are unlikely to meet the strict criteria set for primary imaging tests for implant planning (Reiskin et al 1998).46 In addition, panoramic image cannot provide clinicians with information about the buccolingual cross-sectional dimension or the inclination of the alveolar ridge. Assessments of mesiodistal distance can be very imprecise due to inappropriate patient positioning and/or individual variations in jaw curvature. Therefore, it is of limited value in demonstrating critical structures but is of very little use in depicting the spatial relationships between the structures and dimensional quantification of the implant site.

Fig. 3

Panoramic Radiographs Showing Implant in Position

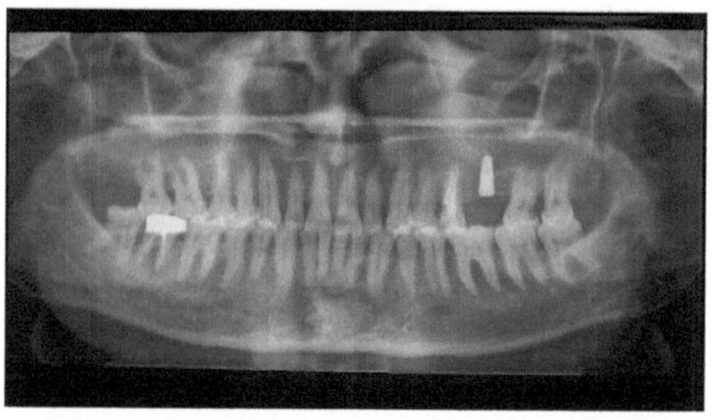

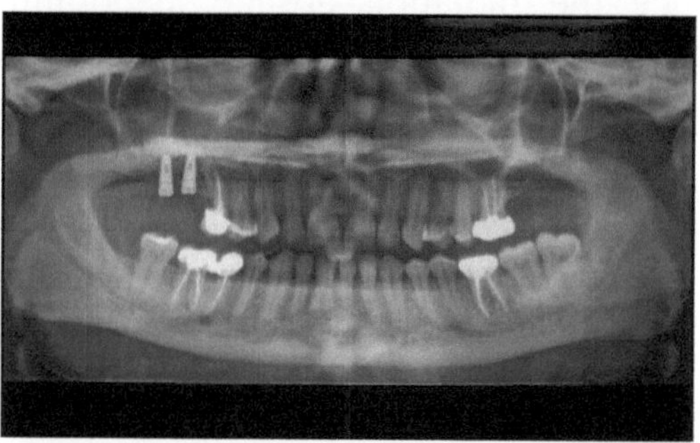

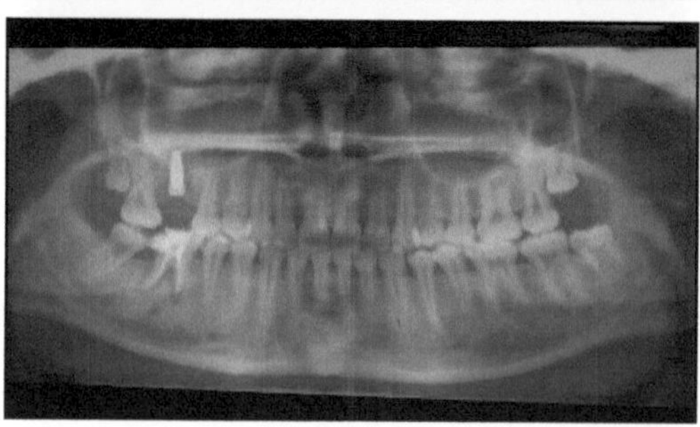

Panoramic Radiographs Showing Implants in Position

C. LATERAL CEPHALOMETRIC RADIOGRAPHY:

Lateral cephalometric radiographs are produced with the patient's midsagittal plane oriented parallel to the image receptor by using a cephalometer. The cephalometer physically fixes the position of the skull with projections into the external auditory canals. Lateral cephalometric radiographs have been recommended for evaluating the anterior maxilla and mandible for dental implant placement. They can accurately measure the height and width of the residual bone at the anterior midline of both the maxilla and mandible. Lateral cephalometric radiography also allows analysis of the quality of the bony host site (ratio of compact to cancellous bone), particularly that in the anterior region of the mandible (Lekholm et al 1985).[47] The soft tissue profile is also apparent on the radiographs and can be used to evaluate profile alterations after prosthodontic rehabilitation (Shetty et al 1999).[44] If a patient is already wearing a denture, a recording should be made with the denture in place in order to provide information about the preoperative relationships between the maxilla and mandible (Strid et al 1985).[42]

Beltrao et al (2007)[45] presented an objective and simple technique that employs a lateral cephalometric radiograph for the preoperative planning of maxillary implant reconstruction with autogenous bone graft. Lateral cephalometric radiographs were performed with a metallic marker placed inside an acrylic-coated model, followed by cephalometric studies, to predict the most adequate grafting method for maxillary reconstruction in 13 edentulous patients (2 males and 11 females) whose age ranged from 27 to 47 years (mean age 37.9 years). It was possible to predict the type of maxillary reconstruction in all patients. Onlay graft was used in 12 patients. One patient was submitted to LeFort I reconstruction with interpositional graft. After 8 months, the patients received a total of 95 standard implants. The success rate was 94.7% with loss of five implants. Rehabilitation was performed with protocol-type prostheses. All patients have been followed for more than 18 months since osseointegration. Authors concluded that this was a simple and objective method provided a useful contribution to maxillary reconstruction, and to the functional and aesthetic rehabilitation of the patients.

Simon et al (2013)[46] highlighted a simple modification that was made to enhance a two-dimensional view provided by a lateral cephalogram to enable placement of a dental implant to replace the missing left maxillary lateral incisor, that was complicated by the presence of a narrow space. An eighteen year old boy with a chief complaint to replace his missing left maxillary lateral incisor. A detailed case history was taken. The investigations revealed that the total mesiodistal space in the region of the missing lateral incisor was 6mm, with adequate length in the cervico apical region as compared to the roots of the adjacent teeth. The ridge mapping procedure revealed that there was adequate bone in the buccolingual dimension to accommodate a mini implant with a diameter of 3 mm diameter The modification was made possible by fabricating an occlusion rim in the region missing maxillary left lateral incisor region and placing a custom made L shaped 21 gauge wire in the space of the missing teeth. The L shape of the wire was initially angulated using the long axis of the adjacent teeth and the inclination of the labial alveolar mucosa and the temporary splint was placed in the maxillary arch to facilitate a lateral Cephalometric radiograph. The resulting image was used to align the L shaped 21 gauge wire to make it lie parallel with the angle formed by the labial alveolar bone in the region of the maxillary left lateral incisor. A second image was then made to confirm that the angle formed by the L shaped wire was coinciding with the angle formed by labial surface of the alveolar bone in the region of the maxillary left lateral incisor. The occlusion rim was then converted to a surgical template with the final L shaped wire embedded into the labial surface adjacent to the missing maxillary lateral incisor. Authors concluded that the modified technique using the cephalogram in addition to the other diagnostic technique proved to be an approximate guide to the surgical procedure.

Lateral cephalometric radiographs offer limited information about the symphyseal area, and the inclination and buccolingual dimensions of the anterior jawbone region. They are not very useful when planning placement of implants lateral to the mid-sagittal plane. Moreover, due to the presence of genial tubercles, lateral cephalometric radiographs may create overly optimistic bone volume assessments (Jacobs et al 1998).[47] With a fixed relationship between focus-film and film-object distance, there is a uniform magnification of about 10% (7-12%) (Shetty et al 1999).[44]

Periapical radiographs produce a high resolution planar image of a limited region of the jaws. Periapical radiographs do not provide any cross-sectional information of the jaws and may suffer from both distortion and magnification. However, the long cone paralleling technique eliminates distortion and limits magnification to less than 10%. Occlusal radiography produces high resolution planar images of the body of the mandible or the maxilla (Kircos and Misch 2005).[27] Cephalometric radiographs are a useful tool for the development of an implant treatment plan, especially for the completely edentulous patient or for placement of implants near the midline for overdentures.

Panoramic radiography is a curved plane tomographic radiographic technique used to depict the body of the mandible, maxilla, and the lower one half of the maxillary sinuses in a single image. This radiographic technique produces an image of a section of the jaws of variable thickness and magnification. The vertical height of bone initially can be assessed. Useful in making preliminary estimations of crestal alveolar bone and cortical boundaries (Benson and Shetty 2009).[3] The procedure is performed with convenience, ease and speed. Accurate assessment of hard tissue morphology and density is difficult because of the variable distortions occurring in different parts of the radiograph (Schwarz et al 1990).[48] Panoramic image cannot provide clinicians with information about the buccolingual cross-sectional dimension or the inclination of the alveolar ridge. Assessments of mesiodistal distance can be very imprecise due to inappropriate patient positioning and/or individual variations in jaw curvature (Langland et al 1989).[49] It is of limited value in demonstrating critical structures but is of very little use in depicting the spatial relationships between the structures and dimensional quantification of the implant site (Kircos and Misch 2005).[27]

CHAPTER 3:
DIGITAL SUBTRACTION RADIOGRAPHY

Subtraction methods were introduced by B. G. Zeides des Plantes in the 1920s. Subtraction radiography was introduced to dentistry in 1980s (Bragger et al 1988, Grondahl et al 1983).[4,50] It was used to compare standardized radiographs taken at sequential examination visits. All unchanged structures were subtracted and these areas were displayed in neutral gray shade in the subtraction image; while regions that had changed, were displayed in darker or lighter shades of gray (Reddy et al 1999).[51] Digital subtraction of images has been applied to dental radiography for more than 20 years. Film subtraction was the established standard method for cerebral angiography and was widely used until digital subtraction fluoroscopy became available in the late 1970s. Nowadays, filmless' photoelectronic imaging systems, especially video fluoroscopy, are used to subtract diagnostic images (Vannier et al 1996).[52] The detection of small changes in serial radiographs using subtraction methods introduced by Zeidses des Plantes is socalled 1st generation of subtraction systems and it employs photographic techniques for the subtraction of a priori registered radiographic films that are aligned manually. The 2nd generation performs digital subtraction by means of computer. One of the earliest methods in dental radiology was reported by GroÈ ndahl et al. in the early 1980s (Grondahl et al 1983).[50] Based on standardized radiographs, the reference (baseline) radiograph is digitized, converted to an exact positive image by the computer and displayed on a television (TV) screen. A TV-camera is then connected to the same screen and the subsequent (follow-up) image in its negative modality is superimposed on the positive reference image. By means of a device permitting rotation and translation of the subsequent radiograph, it is aligned and then digitized. Ortman et al. added a second stage to this manual adjustment procedure where both images are presented sequentially in a "Flicker-mode". Bragger and coworkers suggested the use of three stages to register the images during digitization. Coarse registration is done by a `chessboard'-mode. Numerous studies, starting in the early 1980s, have proven that digital subtraction radiography is capable of exquisite sensitivity to small changes, provided that the experimental conditions can be held constant.

There are two considerable methods in digital fluoroscopy viz. "temporal subtraction" and "energy subtraction"

Comparison of Temporal & Energy subtractions

When the two techniques are combined, the process is called "Hybrid Subtraction". Image contrast is still enhanced further by hybrid subtraction because of reduced patient motion between taking subtracted images. Temporal subtraction techniques are more often used because of limitation of high voltage generators in the energy subtraction techniques. When the two images of the same object are registered and intensities of corresponding pixels are subtracted, a uniform difference image is produced. If there is a change in the radiographic attenuation between the baseline and follow-up examination, this change shows up as a brighter area, when the change represents gain, and as a darker area when, the change represents loss (White et al 2004).[53]

Jung et al (1996)[54]evaluated radiographically alveolar bone loss during the first 12 months after implant abutment connection. Sixty-two implants in 62 partially edentulous patients, aged 17 to 62 years were selected. The subjects included 37 males and 25 females with 24 implants in maxillae and 38 in mandibles. Types of implants used included 17 miniseries, 11 standard series, and 18 hex-lock series from the Steri-Oss Implant System (Steri-Oss, Yorba Linda, CA), as well as 16 3i standard implants (Implant Innovations, West Palm Beach, FL). Changes in bone density were measured by the digital subtraction image radiographic method. At 3-month intervals for 1 year, bone loss around the four types of implants used (standard series, miniseries, and hex-lock implants of the Steri-Oss system; and 3i standard implants) was investigated. Rapid bone loss around all four implant types occurred in the first 3 months. Most of the implants showed resorption of alveolar bone beyond the polished neck at 12 months. The bone level stabilized at the first thread of the implants with no correlation to either the time of exposure of the polished neck or the type of implant. Authors concluded that bone density decreased at the marginal bone and increased at the newly formed alveolar crest.

Kwon et al (2001)[55]assessed thc change of bone density after first, second surgery of dental implant and the amount of marginal bone loss during 9-months after second surgery using digital subtraction radiography. 17 Brånemark implants of 3.75mm in diameter, 2 Brånemark implants of 5.0mm in diameter, 11 ReplaceTM implants of 4.3mm in diameter were included in this study. To standardize the projection geometry of serial radiographs of implants, customized bite block was fabricated using XCP film holder(Rinn Corporation, Elgin, IL.) with polyether impression material of Impregum(ESPE, Germany) and direct digital image was obtained. Qualitative and quantitative changes on radiographs were measured with Emago software (The Oral Diagnostic System, Amsterdam, Netherlands). The peri-implant bone density of 69.2% implants did not change and the peri-implant bone density of 30.8% implants decreased after 3 months following first surgery. The crestal bone density of 53.9% implants decreased first 3 months after second surgery. The crestal bone density of 58.8% implants increased 9 months after second surgery. No density change was observed around the midportion of the implants after second surgery. The amount of marginal bone loss between different kinds of implants showed no statistically significant differences ($p>0.05$). More than 90% of total marginal bone loss recorded in a 9-month period occurred during the first 3 months.

Carneiro et al (2012)[56]assessed longitudinal quantitative changes in bone density around different implant loading protocols and implant surfaces, measured by DSR. 12 patients received bilateral homologous standard and TiUniteH (Nobel Biocare, Kloten, Switzerland) single-tooth implants under 2 implant— loading protocols: immediate loading (8 patients, 16 implants, 12 maxillary) and conventional loading (4 patients, 8 implants, 4 maxillary). Standardized periapical radiographs were taken immediately after implant placement (baseline image) and at the 3-month, 6-month and 12-month follow ups. Radiographic images were digitized and submitted to digital subtraction using the DSR systemH (Electro Medical System, Nyon, Switzerland), resulting in three subtracted images. Quantitative analysis of bone density was performed using Image ToolH software (University of Texas Health Science Centre, San Antonio, TX) to assess pixel value changes in five areas around the implants (crestal, subcrestal, medial third, apical–lateral and apical). Repeated-measures analysis of variance showed that grey levels were significantly influenced by follow-up time and implant-loading protocol. A linear increase in grey levels was found for immediate loading (IML) implants and a significant decrease in grey levels was observed in the 12-month follow up for conventional loading implants. No effect of implant surface treatment was observed. Authors concluded that IML protocol induced mineral bone gain around single-tooth implants after the first year under function for cases with favourable bone conditions and a decrease in bone density around conventional loading implants.

Bittar-Cortez et al (2006)[57] compared hard tissue density changes around implants using digitized conventional radiographs with subtraction image. Thirty-four patients were monitored by standardized periapical radiographs 1 week after surgery and 4 months later. The radiographs were digitized and manipulated by means of EMAGOs software. Linear and logarithmic DSI were obtained, and a filter was added to the logarithmic image. Control and test regions were selected and the mean value of the gray level of the histogram of these selected areas was obtained. This process was carried out in the digitized conventional radiographs (DCR) and the two methods of DSI. After that, the images were divided into two groups, with and without bone loss, and statistical analysis was performed. The results indicate that differences between the jaws did not reach significance, in all the images and in the two groups with and without bone loss. Furthermore, there was no statistically significant difference between the radiographic density assessed in the DCR and the two methods of subtraction images. Author concluded that digitized conventional radiographs and the two methods of digital subtraction images can be used to monitor peri-implant bone density.

Bittar-Cortez et al (2006)[58]compared peri-implant bone level assessment in digitized

Conventional radiographs and digital subtraction images. The bone height around 30 implants in 22 patients was assessed by 5 observers. Standardized periapical radiographs were obtained just after the surgery and 4 months later. The radiographs were digitized and manipulated by means of EMAGOw software, and linear and logarithmic DSIs were produced. Furthermore, the logarithmic subtraction was enhanced with the use of a filter. The observers had the DRs and three methods of subtraction to assess bone height. ANOVA statistical procedures were applied to analyse differences between the observers in the four assessed images and the Tukey test was used to evaluate the differences between the images. Comparison of the bone height assessments indicated significantly (P, 0.05) higher values in the DR than the three methods of DSI. The observers also had a statistically significant variability in this assessment (P = 0.00003).Author concluded that lower values of linear measurements of the bone height around endosseous implants of DSI, compared with DR. Interobserver variability should be considered when comparing values from follow-up studies.

Mehdizadeh et al (2014)[59] compared changes in bone height around endosseous implants using digital conventional radiographs (DCR) with direct digital subtraction images (DSI) prior to loading. In this study, 10 dental implants from 6 patients were studied. Standardized digital radiographs were obtained one week and 3 months postoperatively and subtracted by means of EMAGO software. Then two radiologists evaluated bone height on digital conventional radiographs and digital subtraction images. Data was analyzed with paired t-test using the MINITAB 1.4 software program. Comparative evaluation of bone height indicated significantly higher values on DCR than on DSI (p value = 0.002). The observers also had statistically significant variability in this assessment (p value = 0.00003).Authors concluded that DSI technique can be effective in predicting the dental implant success because it can show lower amounts and fewer differences in evaluation of bone height reported by different operators.

DSR has made a significant improvement in the detection of dental & maxillofacial lesions (Brent et al 2000).[60] With conventional radiography, a change in mineralization of 30-60% is necessary to be detected by an experimented radiologist (Matteson et al 1996)[6] also the lesions restricted to cancellous bone could not be detected because of its less mineral contents than cortical bone (Wengraf et al 1964)[61] but with DSR the alveolar bone changes of 1-5% per unit volume and significant differences in crestal bone height of 0.78 mm can be detected (Sanz et al 2002).[62] Also, defects of at least 0.49mm in depth of cortical bone can be detected whereas a lesion must be at least 3 times larger to be detectable with the conventional radiography techniques (Christgau et al 1998).[8] Furthermore, it can be used to assess the bone at each of three phases of implant treatment, evaluation & maintenance (Reddy and Wang et al 1999).[51] Another application of DSR is in Temporomandibular Joint imaging, esp. with panoramics. The TMJ imaging programs allowed imaging of the right & left mandibular condyles in the open & closed positions on a single film, but the condylar head & intra-articular space were not depicted clearly because of the superimposition of the surrounding structures & the oblique projection of the joint. So, elimination of the superimposed structures with digital subtraction technique improves the visualization of condyle (Masood et al 2002).[63] DSR has also been used in the evaluation of the progression, arrest, or regression of caries lesions. The caries lesions are not well-defined radiolucencies, thus the measurement of their extent is difficult in conventional radiography. In addition it is used for evaluation of endodontically treated teeth (Sun et al 1991).[64] And has the ability to detect root resorption as low as 0.5mm and when underexposed radiographs are used, it can detect even soft tissue changes. So any lesion (including bony cysts or tumors) with potential of change over time can be studied in this technique (Brooks et al 2003).[65] Digital radiography also offers useful advantages in cephalometric analysis and growth prediction of the facial structures. DSR also has a role in research purpose as the nature of digital images itself renders the technique very useful for a variety of scientific research approaches. Since digital images come as pure mathematical information, modern data processing can easily be applied making digital radiography an enormously useful source for scientific purposes.

There are several advantages of DSR such as, Lower dose of radiation: Digital imaging requires lower dose of radiation as compared to conventional radiography. Computer manipulation: Computer manipulation is useful to modify contrast, colour, size of images as well as the visibility of the structures, Image analysis: Automated image analysis may be performed by means of modern data processing. This is a particularly promising feature of digital radiography for the (near) future, No film processing: No need for conventional processing, thereby avoiding all film processing errors and hazards associated with handling the chemical solutions, Time reduction: Digital radiographs are acquired almost in real time (solid state detector systems), Storage: Due to legal requirements in many countries, radiographs have to be stored over a long period of time. Digital radiographs can easily be stored on various digital storage media in a space saving manner. However it should be kept in mind that change in digital file formats and operating systems may pose hazards in opening older files, Easy and quick image transfer, Digital images may be easily and quickly transmitted between institutions or offices, i.e. simply to avoid additional exposure for the patient. Also they have some limitations like Cost: Purchasing digital radiographic systems is expensive, particularly panoramic systems, Storage capacity: The larger the image, the more storage space is required, Handling problems: Rigid direct digital receptors may induce patient discomfort and correct positioning in the hard palate region is beset with difficulties, Loss of resolution: Particularly most storage phosphor systems offer a lower optimal resolution when compared to radiographic film. If at all, however, this may only be relevant for high-resolution intraoral radiography where fine detail such as the tip of a very thin endodontic file has to be visualized, Image manipulation: Digital image may be more easily prone to intentional manipulation. For a successful DSR, reproducible exposure geometry, and also identical contrast and density of the serial radiographs, are essential prerequisites, and long experience shows that this technique is very sensitive to any physical noise occurring between the radiographs (Christgau et al 1998)[8] and even minor changes leads to large errors in results. Hence, the projection geometry and contrast & density should be standardized by a step wedge, to avoid misinterpretation of the subtracted images (Fidler et al 2000).[66] Differences in the image contrast and intensity between the baseline and the follow-up images can hamper the detection task and make the quantitative measurements unreliable .Digital imaging soft-wares commonly include a histogram tool, as well as tools for the adjustment of brightness and contrast. Some tools also allow adjustment of the gamma value. Projection artifacts can be caused by misangulation of the central beam in relation to the film holder and the film. Grondahl showed that angulation discrepancies less than three degrees can produce interpretable subtraction images; Ruttiman et al (2000) reported that angulation errors should be limited to two degrees. Customized occlusal stents can be used to align the film's reproducibility to the dentition. But, stents can be used for a follow up period of less than 2 years and also they can be used in limited number of patients. In 1987, Jeffcoat et al described a method based on the use of cephalostat to maintain the position of the patient's head and a long source-to-object distance (more than 50 inch). In this method, the patient could be reproducibly placed within the cephalostat with less than 0.33 degrees of difference between the exposures and a non-divergent X-ray beam would pass through the patient and will be captured by an intraoral film but cephalostat is expensive and also it needs adequate space to accommodate the long source-to-patient distance.

The digital subtraction radiography technique accommodating a digital dental imaging system should be acknowledged as a reliable method for quantitatively & longitudinal assessing any lesion with a potential of change over time. DSR has made a significant improvement in the detection of dental and maxillofacial lesions, in Temporomandibular Joint imaging and evaluation of the progression, arrest, or regression of caries lesions.

But still there is no definite and accurate simple solution to control projection geometry and correct the discrepancies due to that, so this technique has still not been widely adapted to dental profession and the efforts are underway to solve these problems.

CHAPTER 4:

MAGNETIC RESONANCE IMAGING

For safe implant placement, full knowledge of the shape and quality of the implant site is a prerequisite. Incorrect presurgical assessment can at best lead to implant failure, and at worst to damage to nerves (Berberi et al. 1993; Ellies & Hawker 1993)[67,68] and blood vessels (Ten Bruggenkate et al. 1993),[69] perforation of the maxillary sinus (Regev et al. 1995)[70] and other sequelae. A number of methods for assessment have been developed. Magnetic resonance imaging (MRI) does not use ionising radiation. Instead, the patient is placed in a strong magnetic field and subjected to short pulses of radio waves. MRI is based on the phenomenon of nuclear magnetic resonance (NMR), which was first described independently by two groups of workers in the USA (Bloch et al. 1946; Purcell et al. 1946).[71,72] In the 1950s, NMR was used by chemists to examine molecular structure.

MRI uses signals from hydrogen nuclei (protons) in water and fat to form cross-sectional images of the body. In the USA, Damadian (1971)[73] reported increased hydrogen NMR relaxation times in cancerous tissues, allowing detection of tumours, while Lauterbur (1973)[74] developed the imaging principle which allows us to construct MR images. These initial ideas were developed into a practical imaging tool in the UK. The first clinical whole body scan was performed in Aberdeen (Edelstein et al. 1980; Hutchison et al. 1980),[75,76] while groups in Nottingham and London pioneered brain imaging (Hawkes et al. 1980; Young et al. 1981).[77,78] Redpath (1997) has reviewed the technical development of MRI which followed Lauterbur's 1973[74] paper. MRI has been used in the head for investigation of temperomandibular joints (Katzberg 1989),[79] facial nerve studies (Wortham et al. 1989)[80] and tumour pathology (Wong 1996).[81]

In MRI, to create images, we use a strong uniform static magnetic field, switched magnetic field gradients, with radiofrequency magnetic field pulses (Stark & Bradley 1999).[82] The molecular environment and the proton densities influence the relative intensities of the MR signal produced. The signals from the hydrogen protons in water and fat vary depending on the nature of the tissue being examined. Most MRI magnets operate in the mid-field range (approximately 0.5–1.5tesla, where 1tesla is around 20,000 times the strength of the earth's magnetic field). Mid-field scanners usually require the subject to be imaged within a tunnel, which may cause claustrophobia (Medical Devices Directorate 1993). McIsaac et al. (1998)[83] reported that 25% of participants of their study experienced anxiety during MRI scanning. Novel low-field scanner designs allow the subject to be imaged with an 'open magnet', which offers a less claustrophobic imaging environment. Minor interventional surgery may even be performed in open scanners (Jolesz et al. 2001; Parkkola et al. 2001).[84,85] Spouse & Gedroyc (2000)[86] reported a 94%success rate when scanning a group of patients in an open magnet who had failed to accept a conventional MRI scanner. High-field scanners (above 1.5tesla) which allow very high spatial resolution have been used for dental research on *ex vivo* samples (Lockhart et al. 1992, Baumann & Doll 1997).[87,88] Improvements in MRI technology may allow these techniques to be applied clinically.

MR images are often described as being either T1- or T2-weighted. T1 and T2 refer to the longitudinal and transverse proton relaxation times, respectively. T1- and T2- weighted sequences are made by varying the timings of the radiofrequency pulses, thus altering the sequence repetition time (TR), the echo time (TE) and, hence, image contrast. In general, T1-weighted images are used to show normal anatomy, while T2-weighted images are useful for detection of infection, haemorrhage and tumours. Due to the different information available from T1- and T2-weighted images in neoplastic tissue, both sequences should be obtained when investigating pathology. To reduce the effect of fatty tissue such as cancellous bone making interpretation difficult, the technique of fat saturation may be used. This technique utilises the small difference (3.5 parts per million (p.p.m.) in resonant frequency between protons in water molecules, and those in lipid molecules, to suppress the signal from fat. A review of the principles and clinical applications of MRI may be found in Stark & Bradley (1999).[82]

Aguiar et al (2008)[89] compared the reliability of MRI with CT for dental implant planning with respect to bone measurements. 5 dry human mandibles were submitted for MRI and CT examinations. Each mandible at 3 sites were identified by the markers at the anterior region of each mandible, in a total of 15 sites. The images provided by the MRI and CT examinations were delivered to four specialists in Oral and Maxillofacial Radiology to measure the bone height at the specific sites. Subsequently, the bone height of the dry mandibles was directly measured in the determined sites. The measurements obtained by the specialists in MRI and CT images were compared with the measurements obtained directly from the dry mandibles using the ANOVA test with a 0.05 significance level. The differences between measurements obtained directly from dry mandibles and measurements from the MRI examinations varied from 0.13 to 1.67mm, where 10–15 sites analysed were overestimated in MRI examinations and five were underestimated. The differences between measurements obtained directly from dry mandibles and measurements from the CT examinations varied from 0.02 to 1.25mm, with nine sites being overestimated in the CT examination and six being underestimated. Analysing the measurements obtained from the MRI examinations and those from the CT scans, the differences varied from 0.03 to 1.mm, with nine sites giving higher values in MRI examinations, and six sites giving higher values in CT examinations. The Author concluded that the MRI, when compared with CT, shown to be reliable in respect to bone measurements for dental implant planning.

Gray et al (1998)[90] evaluated the use of a low- field magnetic resonance scanner for assessment of available bone for placement of osseo-integrated dental implants. Eleven patients in which total 19 implants (13 maxillary and 6 mandibular) were placed to assess suitability of implant. A 0.2 tesla low-field 'open' scanner was used for this study. A clear acrylic dental bite registration block was made to act as an imaging template. Holes with 2mm diameter were drilled into acrylic block over potential implant sites and filled with gadolinium markers to allow accurate location of the implant sites. In all cases, clear identication of the inferior dental, mental nerves and the lower border of the maxillary sinus were assessed. The operating confidence was high, and implants can be safely placed in regions, which might be in contention when using other imaging techniques. Artefacts were few and localized, (noted on one site in one case only). The appearance of soft tissues in the scan allowed the surgeon to assess the final profile of the patient. Author concluded that low- field magnetic resonance imaging has definite potential for pre-implant assessment. Full sectional information was readily available at any desired plane with no need for reformatting. The information for accurate and safe implant placement was clear. The technique uses no ionizing radiation.

Gray et al (2001)[91] assessed in this case report magnetic resonance imaging for a sinus lift operation using reoxidised cellulose (Surgicel) as graft material. A 50 year old man was selected for placement of dental implant with 24 having insufficient bone height. Sinus lift procedure was performed by using surgical. At 3 months post operation, a low-field MRI scan was performed, using a 0.2 T ''Open Viva'' magnetic resonance imaging (MRI) scanner by using Magnevist injection. The vertical bone height (from the oral cortical plate to the sinus surface) was measured at three points delineated along the edentulous portion of the arch. As the interface between new and old bone could be clearly delineated, the pre-surgical vertical bone height was measured at the same three points along the arch. Measurements of vertical bone height from the pre-surgical panoramic radiograph were also made at the same horizontal spacing used in the MRI scans. This vertical measurement of the preoperative bone height on the MRI scan was related to the preoperative vertical measurements from the panoramic radiograph. The MRI scan apparently showed a new layer of cortical bone forming below the antral mucoperiosteum. Author concluded that the use of MRI in the examination of healing graft sites was allowed to gain significant information without the use of ionizing radiation, and allows full tomographic examination of the sinus lift region.

Pompa et al (2010)[92] compared magnetic resonance imaging with computed tomography for dental implant planning in respect to bone measurements. 30 patients were selected with monoedentulism or partial edentulism requiring the insertion of osseointegrated implants in which scans were performed with CT and MR. The CT DentaScan was performed for each patient according to standard procedures. The MR of the jaws,for implant evaluation purposes, was performed by acquiring images PD, T2-weighted and Tl-weighted. The measurements obtained by the specialists in MR and CT images were compared using the ANOVA tests with a 0.05 significance level. In all 30 cases examined, MR images appeared perfectly comparable to CT images. The differences between the measurements from the MR and CT exams varied from 0.04 to 1.1 mm with no statistically significant difference (P=O.9).Authors concluded that MR,when compared with CT, Shown to be reliable in respect to bone measurement for dental implant planning .

Imamura et al (2004)[93] compared CT and MRI for their ability to detect the mandibular canals and for the dimensional accuracy of their imaging of the cross-sectional areas in the molar region of the lower jaw, where dental implantation is common.11 female patients were selected having at least one partially edentulous site on the mandible (left or right) in the first and second molar regions. Nineteen sites (right or left) on the edentulous mandible were examined with both CT and MRI. CT and MRI cross sections of the first and second mandibular molar regions where the stent marker was the most clearly imaged were compared from the images of 19 mandibular molar regions in the 11 patients. Dimensional accuracy in the second molar region was also compared. With CT, the canals of the first molar regions were not identified in 11 of 19 sites; however, MRI identified the canals in all 19 sites. Using the kappa index, they found that the inter- and intraobserver identification reliabilities (0.84 and 0.87, respectively) were excellent, especially for MRI. Dimensional positioning of the canal in the second molar region was almost the same with MRI as with CT. Author concluded that MRI was an alternative method for use in diagnosis prior to dental implantation in the mandibular molar region.

Although MR image quality is generally good, as for all imaging modalities, artefacts do occur and should be understood to prevent errors in assessment. In dental MRI, two main problems arise, the first due to patient motion, the second due to in homogeneities in the magnetic field caused by magnetic susceptibility effects.

With ever greater accessibility to MRI scanners, reduction in operating costs, and an increased awareness of the advantages of ionising radiation free sectional imaging, the use of MRI in the field of implant dentistry should become established. In many other medical examinations this is indeed the case. Increased research into magnet technology will in time allow us to develop more sophisticated systems, which will in turn allow faster and even more accurate scanners. Future interventional scanners may allow us image guided implant surgery. Sequential 3D scanning opens up the use of MRI as a research tool, allowing us to gain a unique insight into the field of bone and bone graft behaviour.

For safe and accurate placement of dental implants and associated surgical procedures, accurate planning is essential. Sectional imaging is highly desirable, as even simple implant placement after standard two-dimensional radiographic assessment can lead to a significant lack of understanding of the morphology of the site and associated structures. Whilst ionising radiation dose may be significantly reduced with careful use of CT and other X-ray tomograms, the total absence of radiation is a significant advantage of MRI. This, coupled with the flexibility of plane of acquisition, good soft tissue detail, and the low level of imaging artefacts, mean that MRI should be considered as a first choice for preimplant imaging assessment Furthermore, the absence of ionising radiation allows MRI to be used for sequential postoperative research without exposing the patient to radiation hazard. But there are some limitations of MRI over CT like, if the inferior dental canal is surrounded by sclerotic bone, visualization of the canal is more difficult with MRI as the presence of sclerotic bone results in a low bone marrow signal. The reverse is true for CT, as the presence of sclerotic bone in the mandibular body makes the inferior dental canal more obvious. MRI is not useful in characterizing bone mineralization or as high-yield technique for identifying bone or dental disease as compared to computed tomography.

CHAPTER 5

TOMOGRAPHY

With cross-sectional imaging it is possible to supplement the two-dimensional nature of the mentioned radiographs. Conventional tomography offers information on the buccolingual aspect of the bone at potential implant sites. The location of anatomic structures, such as the mandibular canal, and the bone width can easily be determined. In the last two decades, conventional tomographic machines have been introduced in oral health care. Some extraoral X-ray equipment may also offer possibilities for cross-sectional imaging. The tomographic principle is based on sharply visualizing structures in the focal plane, while blurring all other structures. This is achieved by working with different tomographic movements: linear, circular, spiral, elliptical and hypocycloidal. Complex tomographic movements (e.g. spiral and hypocycloidal) are the most widely used. As for all the aforementioned techniques, reliable image interpretation can only be achieved with an optimal projection geometry. Patient positioning is a critical factor and should allow perpendicular projection of the X-ray beam through the bone at the potential implant site. Dental splints with radiopaque markers aid localization in both buccolingual and vertical dimensions, which optimizes the esthetic and biomechanical aspects in the preoperative plan. Digital tomographic images offer increased image quality by contrast enhancement, reduction of blurring and image manipulation. Further image processing may yield precise information on bone volume and (relative) bone density and help to simulate implant surgery by visualizing the planned implant in relation to the anatomic structures.

For radiographic visualization of the mandibular canal, cross-sectional imaging provides the best information. When comparing computed to conventional tomography (hypocycloidal and spiral) for measuring distances to the canal, CT does not seem more accurate (Lindh et al 1989).[94]Spiral tomography performs better than hypocycloidal tomography as the borders of the canal are better identified with the former technique (Klemetti 1993).[95] The greatest inaccuracy is found when using panoramic images (Lindh and Petersson 1989).[94] For preoperative implant planning, spiral tomography seems recommended, because this technique offers an accurate and reliable method to visualize the jaw bone and the related anatomic structures in the buccolingual aspect (Bou et al 2001).[96] It also leads to less radiation dose than spiral computer tomography in restricted edentulous areas (Bou et al 2001).[96] It is worth mentioning that dose values for spiral tomography with the Cranex Tome (Soredex, Helsinki, Finland)are generally 5O–6O% lower than with the Scanora (Soredex), reaching effective dose levels in the first molar region of O.O6 mSv versus O.l2 mSv in the mandible and O.O4 mSv versus O.O8 mSv in the maxilla (Dula et al 2001).[29] When the jawbone to be implanted is a restricted area being compromised with regard to bone quality, quantity or both, spiral tomography may be the preferred planning tool keeping the ratio dose-cost/ benefit balanced. For more extended areas of compromised jawbone or in very complex situations, working in a true three-dimensional image planning environment is justified (Jacob et al 1998).[47] Therefore, various investigators evaluated the effectiveness of CT, CBCT, Dent scan, spiral tomography, linear tomography, sectional/ trans tomography and interactive computed tomography for planning of dental implant therapy.

A) COMPUTED TOMOGRAPHY:

Clinicians have been diagnosing, treatment planning, placing and restoring dental Implants using periapical and panoramic radiographs to assess bone anatomy for several decades. Two dimensional images have been found to have limitations because of inherent distortion factors and the non-interactive nature of film itself provides. With the advent of technology, CT has lead to a new era of implant imaging. CT enables the evaluation of proposed implant sites and provides diagnostic information that other imaging or combinations of imaging techniques cannot provide. CT has several advantages over conventional radiography. First, CT eliminates the superimposition of images of structures outside the area of interest. Second, because of the inherent high contrast resolution of CT, differences between tissues that differ in physical density but less than 1% can be distinguished; conventional radiography requires a 10% difference in physical density to distinguish between tissues. Third, data from a single CT imaging procedure, consisting of either multiple contiguous or one helical scan, can be viewed as images in the axial, coronal or sagittal planes or in any arbitrary plane depending on the diagnostik task. This is referred to as multiplanar reformatted imaging (Frederiksen, 2009).[97]For a long period of time CT has been the gold standard for pre-implant assessment of the jaws. Modern CT units have extremely fast gantry speeds and generate multiple fan-shaped x-ray beams. As a result multislice CT units have very short examination times and isotropic images can be reformatted in any plane. The scan time using a 16-slice Toshiba CT unit is approximately five seconds for one arch. With appropriate software packages, reformatted images are generated in the panoramic plane and cross-sectional images are generated at right angles to the panoramic plane with intervals of between 1 and 2 mm. The CT pre-implant imaging software is designed to produce life-size images that can be used to assess the available bone, the location of vital structures and to present the images in an easy-to-read format. The individual element of the CT image is called a voxel, which has a value, referred to in Hounsfield units (HU), that describes the density of the CT image at that point. HU also known CT numbers, range from -1000 (air) to +3000 (enamel), each corresponding to a different level of beam attenuation (Benson and Shetty, 2009; Frederiksen, 2009; Resnik et al., 2008).[3,97,2] The density of structures within the image is absolute and quantitative and can be used to differentiate tissues in the region (i.e., muscle, 35–70 HU; fibrous tissue, 60–90 HU, cartilage, 80–130 HU; bone 150–1800 HU) and characterize bone quality (D1 bone, >1250 HU; D2 bone, 750–1250 HU; D3 bone, 375–750 HU; D4 bone, <375 HU) (Misch, 2008).[2]

Jacobs et al (1999)[98] evaluated the predictability of 2D-reformatted CT for implant placement by comparing the pre- and intra- operative findings. They included 100 consecutive (partially or fully) edentate patients (59 females, 41 males, age range 15 ± 74 years, mean 53) who, required CT scanning for pre-operative planning of implant placement in the maxilla or posterior mandible. The number, site and size of the implants, the available bone height and anatomical complications were recorded. The pre-operative planning and the outcome at surgery were compared statistically using a percentage agreement and Kendall's correlation coefficient. It should be noted that although 416 implants were planned, only 395 could be placed. The agreement between the pre-operative and intra-operative data on the number of implants (60%) and their respective sites (70%) was good. Agreement for length of implant (44%) and presence of anatomical `complications' (46%) was poor. Kendall's correlation coefficient (t) was highest for the number of implants (0.8) and their sites (0.81), but lower for the length (0.51) of each implant. The author concluded that Reformatted 2D-CT was reliable for the pre-operative assessment of the number and sites of implants in the jaws. However, 2D-CT was formed to be less predictable for the implant size needed and poor for anatomical complications.

Ekestubbe et al (2003)[99] compared the image quality of a storage phosphor screen (the Digoraw PCT System) with that of conventional film–screen in pre-implant conventional tomography, and to test the effect of dose reduction in the storage phosphor system. The study included 11 patients (7 women and 4 men) who were referred for planning of implant treatment in the posterior part of the mandible and in which, Conventional spiral tomography was performed with storage phosphor image plates (Digoraw PCT) at normal and low doses. Ten observers graded the visibility of anatomical structures of importance for implant planning. A three-step rating scale was used, where -1 = worse, 0 = equal and 1 = better than the reference image. Although image quality was graded as equally good in the majority (59%) of images, the storage phosphor system scored significantly lower than film–screen (- 0.37 vs 0.00, respectively) for all the images. Low dose storage phosphor images were rated significantly lower (- 0.21) than normal dose images (0.00). The Author concluded that in the majority of patients, anatomic structures of importance for implant planning in the posterior mandible are visualized equally well on storage phosphor and film–screen images.

Mraiwa et al (2004)[100] assessed the nasopalatine canal on 2D and 3D CT images, in order to describe its morphology, dimensions, relation to the anterior jaw and occurrence of anatomical variations. The study included 34 consecutive spiral CT scans of the maxilla. The CT scans had been taken as part of a clinical procedure for pre-operative planning of implant placement in the maxilla of 34 consecutive patients (17 males and 17 females). The maxillae investigated were fully or partially edentulous. Spiral CT scan from patients with nasopalatine canal pathology were excluded from the study. Scanning was performed using a standard exposure and patient positioning protocol. 2D and 3D spiral CT images were carefully examined for the location, morphology and dimensions of the nasopalatine canal by two independent observers. A comparison was made between 2D observations and 3D using combined observation strategy (paired t-tests). The nasopalatine canal typically appeared as a canal with a mean (standard deviation (SD)) length of 8.1 (3.4) mm. Its palatal opening was the incisive foramen with a mean (SD) inner of 4.6 (1.8) mm. At the level of the nasal floor often 2 (Y-canal morphology), but sometimes 3 or 4 openings could be observed. In particular cases, the canal showed up as a cylinder with only one nasal opening. The average (SD) maximum width of the nasopalatine canal structure at the level of the nasal floor was 4.9 (1.2) mm. The buccopalatal width of the jaw, anterior to the canal was 7.4 (2.6) mm. Interpretation of canal morphology was significantly different, when comparing 2D image observation with 3D combined observation strategy. However, dimensional measurements of the canal were not significantly different for a 2D and a combined 2D/3D approach. The author concluded that, the nasopalatine canal may show important anatomical variations, both with regard to morphology and dimensions. To avoid any potential complications during surgical procedures such as implant placement, a careful pre-operative observation is required. Cross-sectional imaging may be advocated to determine canal morphology and dimensions and to assess anterior bone width for potential implant placement buccally to the canal.

Mathew et al (2015)[101] evaluated the presence, number, position and distribution of vascular channels (VC) in the mandible by using computed tomography. 30 patients were included in this study with partially and completely edentulous areas consisting of 15 males and 15 females of different age groups who were selected for dental implant procedures based on the inclusion and exclusion criteria. The chosen samples were divided into 3 groups: group A (20-39yrs), group B (40-59yrs) and group C (60-79yrs), 10 patients in each with equal number of male and female patients. Dentascan software program was utilized to analyse the images and personal computer used for measurement purpose. For the evaluation of position of vascular channels, measurements were taken by marking a line, with the measuring icon, from the center of alveolar crest with respect to second premolar, first molar and second molar up to the highest point on the superior border. About 63.3% patients [males:10; females:9] demonstrated the presence of lingual vascular channels with 3 of them showing multiple channels. There was higher percentage distribution of VC in males, when compared to females and most common location of VC was found out to be premolar region (82%). The Author concluded that presence and distribution of vascular channels in the mandible assessed by using computed tomography, provided adequate information, which was necessary for the pre-operative planning of dental implant surgery so as to avoid hemorrhage.

Dantas et al (2005)[102] evaluated the influence of patient positioning on the achievement of axial slices using computed tomography for implant planning, observing the differences in the clinical measurements of bone height and width between standard mandibular position and both upper and lower mandibular position. Ten human dry mandibles were randomly chosen with regard to their other anatomical characteristics. They were made in three gantry positions to simulate changes in patient positioning: (1) parallel to the lower base of the mandible (standard); (2) with a gantry inclination of $+19^0$; and (3) with an inclination of -19^0. One examiner measured the bone height and width at selected sites in the images at three different times. Results were compared with a paired test in SAS 8.02. In relation to bone height, when the jaws were inclined to the inferior direction (gantry angle $+19^0$), there was no statistically significant difference for any region studied.

There was a statistically significant difference for the incisor region, when the jaws were inclined to the superior direction (gantry angle -19^0). With respect to the width of the bone rim, there was a statistically significant difference only for the region of the molars, when the jaw was inclined to the inferior direction and for the region of the canine, when the inclination was to the superior direction. The Author concluded that the differences here in observed did not represent a distortion of CT images, but rather an incorrect indication in the cross-sectional reformatting that, instead of being perpendicular, were oblique in relation to the mandibular base.

Ersoy et al (2008)[103] analyzed deviations in the position and inclination of the planned and placed implants with SLA surgical guides using computed tomography. The study included total 21 subjects (eight females and 13 males; 23 to 67 years old; mean age, 43 – 14 years), who underwent implant placement and were treated with computed-generated SLA surgical guides with inclusion criteria like absence of uncontrolled medical conditions, such as diabetes, smoked <20 cigarettes per day, and ‡3-month healing period after extraction at the surgical site. The Exclusion criteria were uncontrolled diabetes, radiation to the head and neck, and the need to graft bone for the implant recipient site because of inadequate bone volume. Radiographic templates were used for all subjects during CT imaging. After obtaining three-dimensional CT images, each implant was virtually placed on the CT images. SLA surgical guides, fabricated using an SLA machine with a laser beam to polymerize the liquid photo-polymerized resin, were used during implant placement. A new CT scan was taken for each subject following implant placement. Special software was used to fuse the images of the planned and placed implants, and the locations and axes were compared. Compared to the planned implants, the placed implants showed angular deviation of $4.9^0 \pm 2.36^0$, whereas the mean linear deviation was 1.22 ± 0.85 mm at the implant neck and 1.51 ± 1 mm at the implant apex. Compared to the implant planning, the angular deviation and linear deviation at the neck and apex of the placed maxillary implants were 5.31^0, 1.04 mm, and 1.57 mm, respectively, whereas corresponding figures for placed mandibular implants were 4.44^0, 1.42 mm, and 1.44 mm, respectively. The Author concluded that computer-aided SLA surgical guides might be accurate tools for transferring ideal implant position from computer planning to the actual implant surgical phase of treatment. In addition, flapless implant placement was possible with these guides.

Cuijpers et al (2013)[104] determined the spatial resolution and sensitivity of micro- versus nano-CT using standardized samples composed of well defined synthetic microspheres embedded in matrices of varying X-ray absorption coefficients and validated the micro- versus nano-CT technique in vivo. To determine spatial resolution and sensitivity, standardized reference samples containing standardized nano- and microspheres were prepared in polymer and ceramic matrices. Thereafter, 10 titanium-coated polymer dental implants (3.2 mm in Ø by 4 mm in length) were placed in the mandible of Beagle dogs. Both micro- and nano-CT, as well as histological analyses, were performed. The reference samples confirmed the high resolution of the nano-CT system, which was capable of revealing sub-micron structures embedded in radiodense matrices. The dog implantation study and subsequent statistical analysis showed equal values for bone area and bone–implant contact measurements between micro-CT and histology. However, because of the limited sample size and field of view, nano-CT was not rendering reliable data representative of the entire bone–implant specimen. The Author concluded that micro-CT analysis WAS an efficient tool to quantitate bone healing parameters at the bone–implant interface, especially when using titanium-coated PMMA implants. Nano-CT was found to be not suitable for such quantification, but revealed complementary morphological information rivaling histology.

Computed tomographic scanning, which allows exact preoperative analysis of the available bone volume and helps to determine the appropriate position, angulation, number, and length of the planned implants, is highly recommended (Schwarz et al 1990).[48] This modality also gives a high-density resolution, and the soft tissues can also be visualized to some degree. The reformatted CT images provide axial, panoramic, and cross-sectional images that are all cross-referenced to one another (Schwarz et al 1987),[105] allowing rapid correlation of the different views. Computed tomography provides a much more accurate estimate of the position of the mandibular canal than does periapical and panoramic radiography and hypocycloidal tomography. For periapical radiographs, the corresponding figure was 53%, for conventional tomography 39%, and for panoramic radiography 17% (Klinge et al 1989).[106] The anterior mandibular buccal depression is more readily detected on CT scans than on panoramic radiographs (Littner et al 1995).[107] Computed tomographic examinations with reformatted images are the only effective means of evaluating the bone volume present below the maxillary sinuses (Andersson et al 1988).[108]

Computed tomographic images give anatomic structures, such as cortical bone, sharper borders than do spiral tomographic images. These apparently clear borders are the result of the calculated linear attenuation for a voxel, which is the weighted average of all tissues. This effect is called partial volume averaging but may result in unreliable depictions of bone thickness and affect the reliability of measurements.

CT is also of value in assessing the quantity and subjective quality of bone prior to harvesting for a bone graft or ridge augmentation procedure. The limitations of CT include a relatively high radiation dose compared to other imaging modalities, the appropriate software is not always available, the cost of the examination is relatively high and not always rebateable from Medicare, the inferior dental canal is not always shown well and beam hardening artefact or scatter from metal restorations can obscure the regions of interest. Lowdensity structures such as osteoid are generally beyond the resolution of CT units. CT radiographers should be encouraged to scan the patient in a way that optimizes the information obtained and that means orientating the patient to minimize artefact from metal restorations and avoiding gantry tilt wherever possible. The presence of a post in the tooth next to the region of interest or close by may result in too much ''beam hardening'' artefact or scatter to make the scan worthwhile. Computed tomography will not be of value in assessing integration of implants as a radiolucent band is usually present around the implant on CT images, but the location of the implant can be assessed in three dimensions using CT. Computed tomography will not be of value in assessing integration of implants as a radiolucent band is usually present around the implant on CT images, but the location of the implant can be assessed in three dimensions using CT.

B. CONE BEAM COMPUTED TOMOGRAPHY:

Because of higher radiation exposure, higher cost, huge footprint, and difficulty in accessibility associated with CT, CBCT was developed. As the name implies, CBCT generates cone-shaped beams and the images are acquired in one rotation by an image intensifier of flat panel detector, resulting in reasonably low levels of radiation dosage (Arai et al., 1999; Chan et al., 2010).[109,23] During the rotation, multiple (from 150 to more than 600) sequential planar projection images of the field of view (FOV) are acquired in a complete, or sometimes partial arch. Obvious advantages of such a system, which provides a shorter examination time, include the reduction of image unsharpness caused by the translation of the patient, reduced image distortion due to internal patient movements, and increased x ray tube efficiency. However, its main disadvantage, especially with larger FOVs, is a limitation in image quality related to noise and contrast resolution because of the detection of large amounts of scattered radiation. The resolution and therefore detail of CBCT imaging is determined by the individual volume elements or voxels produced from the volumetric data set. In CBCT imaging, voxel dimensions primarily depend on the pixel size on the area detector, unlike those in CT, which depend on slice thickness. The resolution of the area detector is submillimeter. Therefore, the theoretical resolution of CBCT is higher than CT.

The reformatted images of CBCT data result in three basic image types; axial images with a computer generated superimposed curve of the alveolar proccss and the associated reformatted alveolar cross-sectional images and panoramic-like images. Such reformatted images provide the clinician with accurate two-dimensional diagnostic information in all three dimensions. Both CT and CBCT images provide information on the continuity of the cortical bone plates, residual bone in the mandible and maxilla, the relative location of adjoining vital structures and the contour of soft tissues covering the osseos structures (Benson & Shetty, 2009).[3]

Voxel values obtained from CBCT images are not absolute values, like HU values obtained using CT, various methods have been proposed to evaluate the bone density (Naitoh et al2009, 2010; Mah et al 2010).[110,112] HU provide a quantitative assessment of bone density as measured by its ability to attenuate an x-ray beam. To date, there was not any standard system for scaling the grey levels representing the reconstructed values. In a study, (Katsumata et al 2007),[113] the authors found that calculated HU on a CBCT scan varied widely from a range of -1500 to over +3000 for different types of bone. However, after a correction has been applied to grey levels with the CBCT, the HU values are much similar to those one would expect in a medical CT device than to the original grey levels obtained from the CBCT scanners (Naitoh et al 2009, 2010; Nomura et al 2010, Mah et al 2010).[110,111,112] The clinical utility of preoperative implant planning by use of in imaging stent that helps relate the radiographic image and its information to a precise anatomic location or a potential implant site. The intended implant sites are identified by radiopaque markers retained within an acrylic stent which the patient wears during the imaging procedure so that images of the markers will b created in the diagnostic images. The imaging stent subsequently may be used as a surgical guide to Orient the insertion angle of the guide bur and hence the angle of the implant. Generally, nonmetallic radiopaque markers are used in CT and CBCT imaging (Benson & Shetty 2009).[3]

The availability of CBCT is also expanding the use of additional diagnostic and treatment software applications. CBCT permits more than diagnosis, it facilitates image-guided surgery. Diagnostic and planning software are available to assist in implant planning to fabricate surgical models (eg, Biomedical Modeling Inc., USA); to facilitate virtual implant placement,; to create diagnostic and surgical implant guidance stents (eg, Virtual Implant Placement, Implant Logic Systems, Cedarhurst, USA; Simplant, Materialise, Belgium; Easy Guide, Keystone Dental, USA) and even to assist in the computer-aided design and manufacture of implant prosthetics (Nobel Guide/Procera software, Nobel Care AG, Sweden). When those programs are applied, different diameters and length of implants can be 'tried in' before the most optimal one is selected. Furthermore, the placed implant can be assessed from several different viewpoints as well as from three-dimensional view. Moreover, once treatment planning is determined in the computer, it can be saved and applied to surgical sites by means of image-aided template production or image-aided navigation. It is important to note that although computer aided implant placement is a promising technique, the unexpected linear and anguler deviation can be a major concern (Chan et al 2010, Ganz 2008).[23,114]

Patients who are edentulous or who are being considered for multiple implant placement may be best imaged by these techniques. The jaws are aligned so that the acquired axial computed tomographic image slices are parallel to the occlusal plane. These axial images are thin (1-2mm) and overlapping, resulting in approximately 30 axial image slices per jaw. The image information of these sequential axial images can be post processed to produce multi two dimensional images in various planes, using a computer based process called multiplanar reformatting (MPR).

Isoda et al (2012)115 evaluated bone quality with density values using cone-beam computed tomography (CBCT) and correlation between bone density and primary stability of dental implants. Eighteen Straumann implants were inserted into 18 fresh femoral heads of swine. The bone densities of implant recipient sites were preoperatively determined by the density value using CBCT. The maximum insertion torque value of each implant was recorded using a digital torque meter. Immediately after the implant placement, RF measurements were performed using the Osstells Mentor. The RF value was measured four times in four directions (every 90^0) for each implant. RF values were represented by a quantitative unit called the implant stability quotient (ISQ) on a scale from1 to 100. The results were expressed in ISQ and averaged for each implant. The density value ranged from 98 to 902. The mean density value, insertion torque, and ISQ of all implants were 591 ±226, 13.4 ± 5.2Ncm, and 67.1 ±8.1, respectively. Statistically significant correlations were found between bone density and insertion torque (rs¼0.796, Po0.001), bone density and ISQ (rs¼0.529, P¼0.024), and insertion torque and ISQ (rs¼0.758, Po0.001). Author concluded that CBCT examination before implant surgery can be helpful for evaluating bone density and predicting the primary stability of the implant.

Parsa et al (2013)[116] analyzed the correlation between bone volume fraction (BV/TV) and calibrated radiographic bone density (HU) in human jaws, derived from micro-CT and multislice computed tomography (MSCT) and also assessed the accuracy of CBCT in evaluating trabecular bone density and microstructure using MSCT and micro-CT. Twenty partially edentulous human mandibular cadavers were scanned for present study. The mandibles were scanned by three types of CT modalities like MSCT, CBCT and micro- CT. In MSCT scans, the occlusal plane of each mandible was set perpendicular to the floor with zero gantry tilt, whereas in CBCT scans, it was set parallel to the floor according to manufacturer's recommended protocol. The edentulous region of each mandible was located at the center of FOV in CBCT scans. Owing to the large gantry of applied micro-CT mandibles were not sectioned to smaller samples. MSCT HU, micro-CT BV/TV, and CBCT gray value and bone volume fraction of each ROI were derived. Statistical analysis was performed to assess the correlations between corresponding measurement parameters. Strong correlations were observed between CBCT and MSCT density measurements ($r = 0.89$) and between CBCT and micro-CT BV/TV measurements ($r = 0.82$) and Excellent correlation was observed between MSCT HU and micro-CT BV/TV. Bland–Altman analysis showed the bias in measuring BV/TV between CBCT and micro-CT was smaller (4.44/lm) than measuring the density between CBCT and MSCT (154.65HU). The 95% measurement errors was between-21.31 to 30.19 for BV/TV and 29.74–279.56 for density measurement. The differences of CBCT and micro- CT BV/TV measurements were minimal (4.44/lm), suggesting strong agreement. Author demonstrated that the reliability and validity of CBCT in bone quality assessment. However, unlike the bone volume fraction measurement, the accuracy for density measurement was unfavorable. In assessing density using CBCT, the microstructural assessment (BV/TV) was therefore recommended.

Shiratori et al (2012)[117] analyzed the precision of CBCT in human skulls by measuring the volume of buccal bone around dental implants and the height between the implant platform and the first contact of the bone at the buccal wall. Eight edentulous dry human cadaver skulls were randomly numbered from 1 to 8, and after this, according to the bone availability, three to six perforations were made at the anterior region of the maxilla and 31 implants were distributed among the eight skulls. An impression coping was made in order to obtain the skull casts, from which the measurements were taken. A mechanical lathe was used for performing wear on the cast. The buccal bone volume measurement was taken at two points: Measurement A, the most apical point possible, and Measurement B, 5mm away from the apical measurement in the direction toward the implant platform. After the implants were placed in the skull, the CBCT was performed to evaluate the bone thickness and the implant platform height to the first contact with the bone on the buccal side. By means of CBCT image, measurements of the bone wall at three points of the implant were obtained, analyzed and compared with those obtained in the plaster skull casting. The results showed that for the three points of the implants, no statistically significant difference in the measurements was obtained from the plaster model and CBCT images. Author concluded that the CBCT can be considered a precise method for measuring the buccal bone volume around dental implants and in determining the bone height between the implant platform and the first contact with bone at the buccal wall.

Slagter et al (2015)[118] evaluated inter and intraobserver reproducibility of buccal base measurement at dental implants with cone beam computed tomography in the esthetic region. Ten patients with a dental implant in the esthetic zone (regions 13 to 23) were included in this study. The CBCT scans were made with an iCAT 3D exam scanner (KaVo Dental GmbH, Biberach, Germany), which was validated for measuring bone thickness. The standard used voxel size was 0.30 and FoV was 100 × 100 mm on the CBCT scans. Bone measurements at implants on the CBCT scans was done using 3D image diagnostic and treatment planning software. Using a new method, buccal bone thickness was measured on ten CBCTs at six positions along the implant axis. Inter- and intraobserver reproducibility was assessed by repeated measurements by two examiners. Mean buccal bone thickness measured by observers 1 and 2 was 2.42 mm (sd: 0.50) and 2.41 mm (sd: 0.47), respectively. Interobserver intraclass correlation coefficient was 0.96 (95% CI 0.93 to 0.98). The mean buccal bone thickness of the first measurement and the second measurement of observer 1 was 2.42 mm (sd: 0.50) and 2.53 mm (sd: 0.49), respectively, with an intraobserver intraclass correlation coefficient of 0.93 (95% CI 0.88 to 0.96). The mean buccal bone thickness of the first measurement and the second measurement of observer 2 was 2.41 mm (sd: 0.47) and 2.52 mm (sd: 0.47), respectively, with an intraobserver intraclass correlation coefficient of 0.96 (95% CI 0.93 to 0.97). Author concluded that CBCT was suitable for reliable and reproducible measurements of buccal bone thickness at implants.

Ibrahim et al (2013)[119] evaluated the accuracy of cone beam CT for trabecular bone microstructure measurement in comparison with micro CT (μCT). Twenty-four human mandibular cadavers were scanned using a CBCT system (80 lm) and a μCT system (35 μm). To obtain the highest spatial resolution possible of an isotropic 80 lm, the smallest field of view (FOV), that is, 4 9 4 cm with the high-resolution scan mode and 360° arm rotation were the selected scan settings. Images were acquired at 90 kV and 5.0 mA. The cadavers were then scanned using a μCT system. Three bone microstructural parameters trabecular number (Tb.N), thickness (Tb.Th) and separation (Tb.Sp) were assessed using CT imaging software. Intraclass correlation coefficients (ICC) showed a high intra-observer reliability (0.996) in all parameters for both systems. The Pearson correlation coefficients between the measurements of the two systems were for Tb.Th 0.82, for Tb.Sp 0.94 and for Tb.N 0.85 (all P's<0.001). The Bland and Altman plots showed strongest agreement in Tb.N (-0.37 μm) followed by Tb.Th (1.6μm) and Tb.Sp (8.8μm).Author concluded that the CBCT system (3D Accuitomo 170) using the highest resolution provides reliable and accurate trabecular bone microstructure measurements when compared with μCT.

Fienitz et al (2011)[120]compared the accuracy of CBCT with histomorphometric measurements in terms of configuration of the buccal bone wall and peri-implant bone regeneration after GBR in animal. Titanium implants were inserted into standard box-shaped defects in the mandible of 12 dogs. Defects of one side were augmented following the principle of GBR, while the other side was left untreated. Radiological evaluation was performed using CBCT and compared with the histomorphometrical measurements of the respective site serving as a validation method. Non - augmented control sites providing a horizontal bone width of < 0.5 mm revealed a significantly lower accuracy between the radiological and the histological evaluation of the buccal defect depth comparing with the group providing > 0.5 mm. In GBR treated defects, the subgroup < 0.5 mm revealed a significantly higher difference between CBCT and histology compared with > 0.5 mm. However, a radiological discrimination between original bone, integrated and non integrated bone substitute material was not reliable. Additionally, it was found that a minimum buccal width of 0.5mm was necessary for the detection of bone in radiology. Therefore, author concluded that peri-implant bone defects regeneration by means of CBCT was not accurate for sites providing a bone width of <0.5mm.

Kamburoglu et al (2014)[121] investigated the accuracy of cone beam CT images in the assessment of buccal marginal alveolar peri-implant defects at different field of view (FOV). Simulated buccal defects were prepared in 69 implants inserted into cadaver mandibles. Implants were randomly inserted into pre-molar and molar regions of denuded cadaver mandibles by an experienced operator. Implants were placed close to the buccal aspect of the mandible to facilitate creation of artificial defects in the buccal cortical marginal alveolar bone. Mandibles were then separated by a bone saw into equal smaller sections, each one comprising two or three implants, and 1.5 cm of wax was applied to the mandibular sections as a soft tissue equivalent material. CBCT images at three different fields of view were acquired: 40 ×40, 60×60 and 100 ×100 mm. The presence or absence of defects was assessed on three sets of images using a five-point scale by three observers. Observers also measured the depth, width and volume of defects on CBCT images, which were compared with physical measurements. All observers had excellent intra-observer agreement. Defect status (p,0.001) and defect size (p,0.001) factors were statistically significant. Pairwise interactions were found between defect status and defect size (p50.001). No differences between median true-positive or true-negative values were found between CBCT field of views (p.0.05). Significant correlations were found between physical and CBCT measurements (p,0.001). Author concluded that all CBCT images obtained at different FOVs with voxel resolutions,0.3mm performed similarly in the detection of simulated buccal marginal alveolar peri-implant defects. In addition, depth, width and volume measurements of the defects from CBCT images correlated highly with actual physical measurements.

Corpas et al (2011)[122] assessed peri-implant bone tissue by comparing outcome of intraoral radiograph with cone beam computed tomography and histological observation. Ten Gottingen male mini-pigs were used as experimental animals. A total of 80 implants were placed in the upper and to the lower jaw. In each of the four quadrants, the last premolar and the first molar were extracted 3 months before the start of the study. To assess matching between different image modalities, measurements conducted on intra-oral digital radiographs (IO), cone beam computer tomography (CBCT) and histological images were correlated using Spearman's correlation. Paired tests (Wilcoxon test) were used to determine changes in the bone parameters after 2 and 3 months of healing. The results showed statistically significant correlations in the bone defect depth between intraoral radiographic images and histological slices (r¼0.7, Po0.01) as well as between CBCT images and histological slices (r¼0.61, Po0.01) .However, intra-oral radiographs and CBCT images yielded a bone defect depth mean underestimation of 1.17 and 1.2mm, respectively, compared with the histological slices. Higher marginal bone levels (>1.5mm) on histological images accounted for higher mean deviations on intra-oral (2.27mm) and CBCT images (2.16mm) when compared with lower (<1.5mm) marginal bone levels (-0.002 and 0.04mm deviation on intra-oral and CBCT images, respectively). For the peri-implant bone fraction, a weak and non significant correlation was found between the mean results obtained on CBCT and on histological images. When monitoring changes over time using intraoral radiography, 2- and 3-month evaluation periods allowed visualizing the peri-implant marginal bone level and density changes, with a significant peri-implant bone loss as established by a more apical position of the marginal bone level after 2 months (1.49mm) and 3 months (1.82mm) of healing compared with the baseline bone level (0.26mm). Author concluded that this study allowed linking radiographic bone defect depth to the histological observations of the peri-implant bone.

Minute bone changes during a short-term period can be followed up using digital intra-oral radiography. Radiographic fractal analysis did not seem to match histological fractal analysis. CBCT was not found to be reliable for bone density measures, but might hold potential with regard to the structural analysis of the trabecular bone.

Zhang (2015)[123] evaluated the alveolar ridge dimension and presence and size of buccal undercut at the maxillary anterior region using cone beam computed tomography for immediate implant treatment planning. A total of 51 subjects with full dentition at right maxilla were included in the study. There were 20 males and 31 females, with an age range of 16–80 years old. CBCT scans were screened and Measurements were taken at the cross sectional views in the middle of the maxillary right central incisor, lateral incisor, and canine regions. Alveolar height was measured from the alveolar crest to floor of nasal fossa. Alveolar width was measured from the buccal to palatal cortical plate at the coronal, middle, and apical third of the distance from the alveolar crest to floor of the nasal fossa. Absence or presence of buccal undercut was demonstrated in a right maxillary canine and a right maxillary lateral incisor. The buccal undercut depth was measured from the deepest point of the undercut at the buccal plate to a line tangent to the buccal plate paralleling the long axis of ridge. Alveolar width increased from coronal to apical direction for each tooth. Mean alveolar widths (mm) were: central incisor, 9.55; lateral incisor, 8.30; canine, 9.62. The lateral incisor had a significantly smaller alveolar width than the other anterior teeth. No significant difference in ridge height was noted among the teeth. Undercut locations from the alveolar crest (mm) were: central incisor, 5.84; lateral incisor, 3.59; canine, 5.11. Undercut depths (mm) were: central incisor, 0.76; lateral incisor, 0.87; canine, 0.73. The percentages of teeth with buccal undercuts were: central incisor, 41 %, lateral incisor, 77 %, and canine 33 %. Male demonstrate significant larger ridge width compared with females for all three teeth. Author concluded that an average alveolar dimension at anterior maxilla is approximately 18 ~ 19 mm in height and 8 ~ 9 mm in width for the selected population and Careful treatment planning with CBCT was critical for successful implant placement, especially at the lateral incisor region due to limited availability of alveolar bone.

Janner et al (2011)[124] analyzed the thickness and the anatomic characteristics of the Schneiderian membrane using cone beam CT in patients for dental implant placement in the posterior maxilla. For the present study, all partially edentulous patients scheduled for limited CBCT imaging for further radiographic evaluation of a future implant insertion site in the posterior maxilla (first premolar to second molar) were consecutively enrolled. Patients with a history of previous dental implant placement or bone grafting in the posterior maxilla, reduced sinus visibility in the CBCT scan volume (less than the region of the anterior maxillary sinus border to the second molar in the sagittal slices; floor of the nose and/or onset of the zygomatic process not visible in the coronal slices), or with evident artifacts due to movement during image taking were excluded from the present study. The study included 143 consecutive patients referred for dental implant placement in the posterior maxilla. A total of 168 CBCT images were taken using a limited field of view of 4 × 4cm, 6 × 6 cm, or 8 × 8 cm. Reformatted coronal CBCT slices were analyzed with regard to the thickness and characteristics of the Schneiderian membrane in nine standardized points of reference. Factors such as age, gender, or status of the remaining dentition that could influence the dimensions of the Schneiderian membrane were evaluated using univariate and multivariate linear regression models. The thickness of the Schneiderian membrane exhibited a wide range, with a minimum value of 0.16mm and a maximum value of 34.61 mm. The highest mean values, ranging from 2.16 to 3.11 mm, were found for the mucosa located in the mid-sagittal regions of the maxillary sinus. The most frequent mucosal findings diagnosed were flat thickenings of the Schneiderian membrane (62 positive findings, 37%). For the multivariate linear regression model, only gender had a statistically significant influence on the mean overall and mid-sagittal thickness of the sinus mucosa. Author concluded that in comparison with CT, modern CBCT devices have the advantage of administering less radiation to the patient. Therefore, CBCT can be regarded as an alternative to CT for three-dimensional imaging before SFE.

Lana et al (2012)[125] evaluated the presence of anatomic variations and lesions of the maxillary sinus in cone beam CT of the maxilla for dental implant planning. They evaluated a sample of 500 consecutive CBCT exams made in a private dental radiology clinic. The CBCT exams were independently evaluated by two oral and maxillofacial radiologists who assessed the presence of anatomic variations and lesions of the maxillary sinus. As most of the CBCT exams did not allow the evaluation of the area close to the maxillary sinus roof, anatomic variations that take place at these sites were not assessed. The anatomic variations detected were pneumatization (83.2%), antral septa (44.4%), hypoplasia (4.8%), and exostosis (2.6%). The identified lesions were mucosal thickening (≤3 mm in 54.8% and >3 mm in 62.6%), polypoid lesions (21.4%), discontinuity of the sinus floor (17.4%), air fluid level (4.4%), bone thickening of the maxillary sinus wall (3.8%), antroliths (3.2%), discontinuity of the sinus lateral wall (2.6%), sinus opacification (1.8%), and foreign body (1.6%).Author concluded that anatomic variations and lesions of the maxillary sinus could be observed in CBCT of the maxilla required for dental implant planning. As some of these conditions can modify dental implant planning and must require specialized treatment, its recognition is noteworthy in dental practice, and especially in implantology.

Fornell et al (2012)[126] presented a simplified technique for CBCT-guided osteotome sinus floor elevation technique for the installation of one to three implants. A total of 14 patients with a total of 21 implants (seven women and seven men; age-range 34–75 years) were included in the study. All patients had reduced bone volume because of vertical bone loss of the alveolar processes and/or extensive pneumatization of the maxillary sinuses. The inclusion criteria were (1) atrophy of the posterior maxilla but with sufficient bone height remaining for primary implant stability at the time of surgery, (2) absence of maxillary sinus disease and (3) absence of pathology affecting neighboring teeth. Preoperative CBCT with a titanium screw post as an indicator at the intended implant position was used to visually guide the flapless surgical procedure. Twenty-one implants all with a length of 10mm and a diameter of 4.1 and 4.8mm were inserted and followed clinically and with CBCT for 3, 6 and 12 months postoperatively. Intraoral radiographs were taken for comparison. All patients were provided with permanent prosthetic constructions 8–12 weeks after implant surgery. The mean height of the residual alveolar process at the time of implant placement was 5.6mm (SD 2.1mm) . The residual bone varied between 2.6 and 8.9mm. Two implants were inserted in 2.6– 2.9mm of residual bone, eight implants were inserted in 3–4.9mm of residual bone, and 4 implants were inserted in 5–6.9mm of residual bone. The remaining seven implants were inserted in 7–8.9mmof residual bone. The mean distance mesial, distal, buccal and lingual was 2.1mm (SD 1.7mm) and varied between 0 and 5.7mm. Corresponding recalculated values for mean vertical apical–intrasinus bone distances were 1.4mm with range 0 and 5.2 mm. The mean sinus elevation was 4.4mm (SD 2.1mm) with range 1.1 and 7.4mm. The mean bone gain was 3mm (SD 2.1mm) with range 0 and 7mm. The mean bone gain as percent of the sinus elevation was 63.3% (SD 28.2%) and varied between 2.3 and 100%.Eighty to 100% bone gain was attained in 33.3% of the implants. Sixty to 79.9% bone gain was attained in 23, 8% of the implants. 42.8% of the implants gained 60% bone of the initial sinus elevation. Author concluded that flapless transalveolar sinus lift procedures visually guided by preoperative CBCT can successfully be used to enable placement, successful healing and loading of one to three implants in residual bone height of 2.6–8.9mm. There was no marginal loss of bone during the 3– 12 months follow-up verified by CBCT.

Apostolakis et al (2011)[127] analyzed the variation in the presence and extent of the anterior loop of the inferior alveolar nerve using CBCT. 320 CBCT consecutive scans were obtained from 320 patients for various clinical indications such as implant planning, trauma, assessment of impacted teeth, etc. using a Newtom VG CBCT device in a private radiological practice for the measurements of the anterior loop length (ALL). The first selection criterion (the border of the mandible depicted) was satisfied by 101 volumes. Of these 101 volumes, five were excluded due to pathology affecting the image (one implant in mental foramen, one osteoradionecrosis, one giant cell lesion, one dense bone island, one artefact due to gunshot pellets). Furthermore, three volumes were excluded due to motion artefacts that rendered the images non-diagnostic. Therefore 93 volumes, representing 93 different patients, were available for evaluation. Using the multiplanar capabilities of the device's software, the prevalence and length of the anterior loop was assessed. The results showed that an anterior loop could be identified in 48% of the cases with a mean length (range) of 0.89 mm (0–5.7). Author concluded that in almost half of the surveyed cases an anterior loop was present. Even though in 95% of the study cases, the loop was <3 mm, a 100% safety margin in the placement of anterior mandibular implants, in the absence of a CBCT scan, would only be achieved with a distance of 6 mm between the anterior border of the mental foramen and the most distal interforaminal implant fixture.

Correa et al (2013)[128] compared the implant size (width and length) planning with digital panoramic radiographs, CBCT generated panoramic views, or CBCT cross-sectional images, in four implant systems. Seventy-one patients requiring single-unit implant(s) in the upper premolar and/or lower molar regions, were included in the study. A total of 103 implant sites were evaluated (43 patients with one implant site, 25 patients with two implant sites, two patients with three implant sites, and one patient with four implant sites). For each patient, digital panoramic radiographs (D-PAN) and CBCTs were recorded. A 5-mm diameter metal ball was fixed by a piece of wax at the intended implant site(s). After acquisition, images were saved as original bitmap format (BMP). CBCT was performed with the ICat New Generation. The unit was set to 120 kV, 5 mA, using a 16 × 6 cm FOV, with an acquisition time of 26.0 sec and a 0.2 mm voxel size. All images were displayed on a monitor and assessed by three observers, who outlined a dental implant by placing four reference points at the site of the implant-to-be placed. Differences in width and length of the implant-to-be from the three modalities were analyzed. The implant size selected in the CBCT-cross images was then compared to that selected in the other two modalities (D-PAN and CBCT-pan) for each of the implant systems separately. The result showed that the implant-to-be (average measurements among observers) was significantly narrower when measured in CBCT-cross compared with both D-PANs and CBCT-pan images. For premolar sites, the width also differed significantly between D-PAN and CBCT-pan modalities, i.e., CBCT-pan allowed wider implants. This was not the case for molar sites. The implant-to-be was also significantly shorter when recorded in CBCT-cross than in D-PAN images. It mattered very little for the change in implant step sizes whether CBCT-cross was compared to D-PAN or CBCT-pan images. Author concluded that selected implants size differs when planned on panoramic or cross-section CBCT images. In most cases, implant size measured in cross-section images was narrower and shorter than implant size measured in a panoramic images or CBCT- based panoramic view.

Suomalainen et al (2008)[129] compared the accuracy of linear measurements in the posterior mandible using dental cone beam CT (3D Accuitomo) with multislice CT (MSCT) by altering the radiation doses during pre-operative planning of oral implant sites. The cadaver mandible was imaged with the CBCT and MSCT devices (i) dry and, in order to better resemble the clinical situation concerning the radiation attenuation and scattering properties of the region examined in patients, (ii) immersed in sucrose liquid isointense with soft tissue (ICRU-44; 53.3 HU) placed in a 1561569 cm plastic box. Low-dose MSCT examinations were performed only with the cadaver mandible immersed in sucrose solution. The position of the mandible in the sucrose solution was maintained at a constant during the examinations. The same human cadaver mandible was used in a previous study to evaluate the accuracy of cross-sectional tomograms obtained with four panoramic radiographic units in the assessment of implant site measurements. Two readers measured four linear distances twice from each section. The mandible was cut into 4 mm slices at the positions marked by the orthodontic tubes. These slices were micro radiographed, measured from the film using a slide gauge and used as the gold standard for measurements. The mean ME for the material as a whole was 6.5%. This varied according to the imaging method. Radiation dose had a significant negative correlation with ME (r520.159, P50.008, Figure 3) as well as with its transformed value (r520.171, P50.004). ME showed significant differences between the methods studied (P50.022). ME was 4.7% for CBCT and 8.8% for MSCT of the dry mandible, 2.3% and 6.6%, respectively, for the mandible immersed in sucrose solution and 5.4% for low-dose MSCT. Lowering the MSCT radiation dose to less than a quarter of its conventional original value did not significantly affect the ME. Author concluded that CBCT is a reliable tool for implant planning measurements compared to MSCT. In this study, a considerable radiation dose reduction could be achieved in MSCT with low-dose settings compared with values obtained for conventional MSCT protocols without adversely affecting measurement reliability.

Typical computed tomographic studies provide information on the continuity of the cortical plates, residual bone in the maxilla and mandible, the relative location of adjoining vital structures, and the contour of soft tissues covering the osseous structures. Reformatted images from CBCT data have been shown to be of equivalent measurement accuracy as MDCT data. These reformations are useful in planning augmentation procedures such as a sinus lift and can provide an estimate of the internal density. A three-dimensional image can provide a visualization of the overall morphology of the intended implant site. Metallic restorations can cause streak artifacts but this can be avoided by aligning the jaws so that the acquired axial scans are parallel to the occlusal plane. CBCT is developed to maxillofacial area to scan and visualize jaw bone lesions especially cancellous bone. This technology offers the surgeon precise views of preplanned locations in the patient's jaw. It is perhaps, when employed as a means for developing surgical guides for implant dentistry that, cone beam CT scanning finds one of its best uses and helps in accurate transfer of preoperative plan to the patients.

Fig. 8

Cone Beam Computed Tomographic Images (CBCT) Showing Pre-Operative and Post-Operative Assessment of Implants

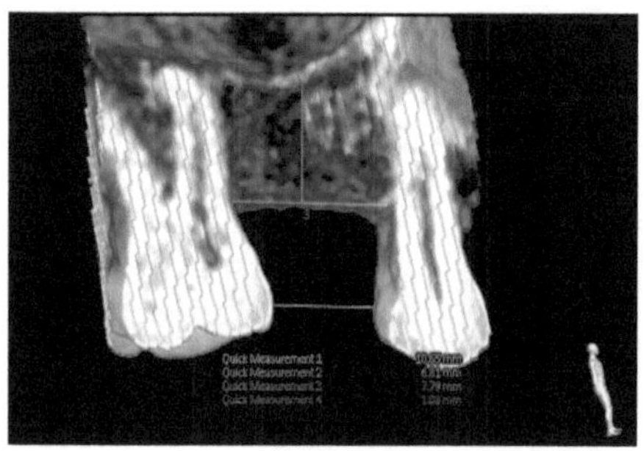

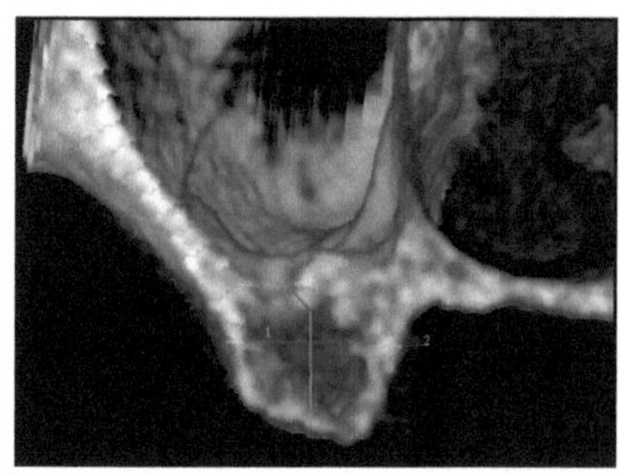

Pre-Operative Assessment of Apical-Coronal Height of Implant Site

Pre-Operative Assessment of Bucco-Palatal Width and thickness of buccal plate

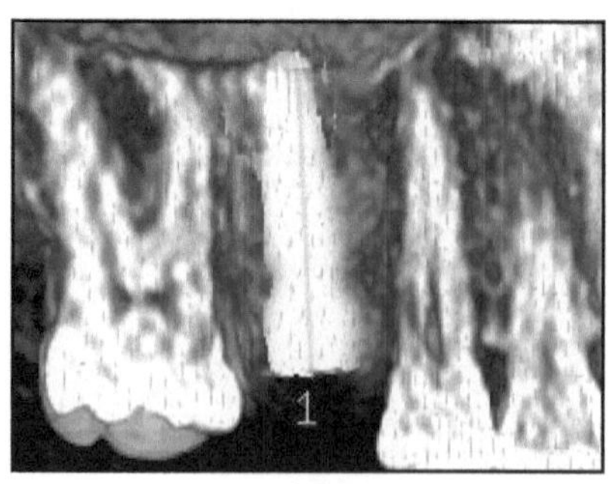

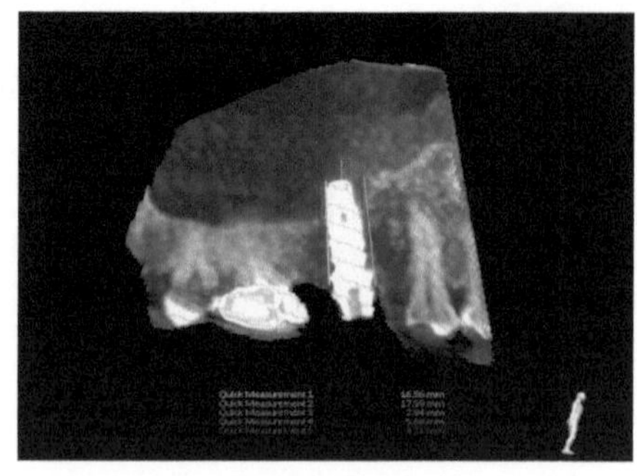

Post -Operative Assessment of Implant Site

D. DENTASCAN :

DentaScan is a unique new computer software program which provides computed tomographic (CT) imaging of the mandible and maxilla in three planes of reference: axial, panoramic, and oblique sagittal (or cross-sectional). The clarity and identical scale between the various views permits uniformity of measurements and cross-referencing of anatomic structures through all three planes. Unlike previous imaging techniques, the oblique sagittal view permits the evaluation of distinct buccal and lingual cortical bone margins, as well as clear visualization of internal structures, such as the incisive and inferior alveolar canals.

A Dentascan examination is a specialized type of computed tomography study (CT or "CAT" scan), which is performed on a conventional CT scanner used to obtain true cross-sections of the mandible and maxilla from the easily obtained CT scans for patients with cyst, tumours, distractions, accuracy of root canal obturation, jaw growth, stages of tooth development, dental implant, cases of fractures in either the mandibular or maxillary arch (Ken Yanagisawa et al 2006).[130]

`Dentascan is used in advanced computer programs to analyze an X-ray study by providing detailed two-dimensional and three-dimensional images and enable nearly diagnosis and plan the details of the surgery with accuracy, well before the operation. Routine dental x-rays are two-dimensional; they only show the location of the teeth and the height of the bone. These x-rays are often distorted, and they cannot depict the thickness of the jawbone; while a Dental CT Scan, on the other hand, is distortion free. It illustrates the actual make-up of the bone and provides three- dimensional and cross-sectional views of the jaws. The life-sized images allow to accurately measure the amount and density of bone (Azari et al 2008).[131]

Jaju et al (2011)[132] examined the multi-planar assessment of maxilla and mandible for implant placement by Dentascans. In twenty five patients were included for this study. The CT scan machine used for this study was Siemens Somatom Sensation 64. This has multidetector (MDCT) technology with 32 detector array and 64 data channels. Dental software used was Syngo Dental CT 2006 A-W VB20B-W. Dental CT slice was of 0.75 mm with reconstruction increment of 0.5 mm, along with an effective mAs of 90 and 120 kilovoltage. Image acquisition of 64 × 0.6 mm with rotation time of 1 s and slice collimation and width of 0.6 mm and 0.75 mm, respectively. Axial, paraxial and panoramic images obtained were evaluated for available ridge height and width at implant sites, proximity to maxillary sinus and inferior alveolar canal, easy identification of inferior alveolar canal, radiographic presence of bony concavities and density at implant sites. Dentascan was an effective software in pre-evaluation of available height and width at the implant sites. There was a co-relation between the available bone at the implant sites and region of jaw, sex and age of patients. Proximity to maxillary sinus and inferior alveolar canal was clearly demonstrated by Dentascans. Inferior alveolar canal was identified in 85.71% cases. Bony concavities were identified in 22.95% cases. Dentascans provide subjective evaluation of bone density in Hounsfield units (symbol HU). Therefore, Author concluded that Dentascans was a rapid, time saving, effective, safe and indispensable procedure in dental implantology.

Dentascan is a great contribution to address surgery, encouraging long term success. Through the DentaScan, a series of axial slices are generated and stored by the radiologist on his computer. These slices are converted by the dentascan radiology module and then copied on to the CD – Rom to be sent immediately to the surgical specialist. Denta Scan networks the axial slices to show three different slice types per screen: axial, panaromic and sectional. Denta scan allows a much faster, easier, efficient and precise study of the CAT scan. Real axial slices will usually be around 1mm, with the option of the even smaller slice parameters (0.5mm). Denta scan generates up to 32 panaromic images showing the mandibular canal and allowing the highlighting of the mental nerves path (visible both in the panaromic and sectional slices) and enabling the detection of some dental pathologies (Klemetti et al 1994).[133]It offers great reassurance to the patients'. 3D simulation offered by Dentascan will make them feel much secure during the surgery.

In case of improper positioning of the patient, the panaromic curve can be reformatted, thus avoiding having to repeat the scan. Information in the slices is reworked to display three different perspectives: axial, panaromic, and sectional, obtaining 3D data. Multiple sectional images enable visual inspection of the cortical thickness, bone trabeculation, intrabony defects, mental nerve location highlighted in the panaromic slice. Maxillary and mandibular evaluation is done: bony defects, impacted roots, hypertrophy of sinus mucosa, sinusitis, deviation of the nasal septum, nasal cornets conditions. A list of bone densities can be generated. All surgical planning can be printed and taken into the operatory.

In difficult cases Denta Scan is being used as an diagnostic tool in treatment planning and identification of several important issues like: Revealing difficulty to detect pathology, Correct assessment of bone trajectory,to avoid iatrogenic injury, Use of CT Scan / surgical template to relate tooth to bone relation, Choosing appropriate implant shape to fit in residual bone.

USES:

- ❖ It allows the visualization of internal bone morphology in three dimensions; therefore the dental surgeon can plan his treatment precisely.

- In cross sectional view, observation regarding bone quality, density can be made typically by direct measurement, if they are present in life size format.
- The main use of dentascan today is in the pre-operative planning and pre-operative modeling of endosseous dental implants and subperiosteal implants (Karl et al 1997).[134]
- It enables the dental surgeon to visualize the bony structures pre-operatively; he does not have to make decisions at the time of surgery when the mucoperiosteal flap is already elevated to visualize the bony structures directly.
- Dentascan CT provides the surgeons an operation with information of the internal structures that cannot even be gained by direct intra-operative visualization. It can also be used for the evaluation of cysts, tumors, and fractures in the jaw (Chidiac et al 2002).[135]
- In the mandible, the precise location of the mandibular canal is critical (Klemetti et al 1994).[133]
- For the maxilla, the location of the floor of the maxillary sinuses is necessary.
- It is important to understand that the anatomy of these bones and surrounding structures is unique to each patient (Yanagisawa et al 2006, Azari et al 2008)[130,131]

LIMITATIONS:

Images may not be of true size and may require compensation for magnification. Determination of bone quality requires use of the imaging computer/ workstation. Hard copy Dentascan images only include a limited range of the diagnostic gray scale of study; and the tilt of the patient's head during the examination is critical because all the cross-sectional images are perpendicular to the axial imaging plane.

E. SPIRAL TOMOGRAPHY:

Spiral tomography was constructed as a multifunctional unit able to meet most dentomaxillofacial radiology needs. Spiral tomography can be performed with the Scanora (Soredex, Orion Corporation Ltd., Helsinki, Finland) which produces buccolingual crosssectional tomograms. Optimal tomographic images can be achieved by using spiral movements where the blurred shadows are placed at equal distances from each other in the partial attenuation zone and when the dose per turn is constant. A panoramic scout image is taken and the regions to be examined are defined. A specific computer program is used for each region of the maxilla or mandible. This system uses a fixedprojection angle to produce a series of four images, 4 mm in thickness, centered 4 mm apart to includc a 16-mm scction of thc jaw on onc film 21. It is possible to obtain four exposures per film using a field size of 7 cm × 10.2 cm. The Scanora has a constant magnification factor of 1.7 (Tammisalo et al 1992)[136] and themachine's slice thickness can be either 2 or 8 mm. When the canines are being examined, it is better to use a 2-mm cut in order to better demonstrate the anatomy in such a curved area. In a study of the reliability of spiral tomography, the inter-observer variations between the first and the second measurements were 1.67 mm and 1.42 mm, respectively; and the corresponding intra-observer variations were 1.07 mm and 0.86 mm. This variability was less than that seen when using hypocycloidal tomography because of the reduction in intra-observer variation and better image quality (Grondahl et al 1991).[137]

Cavalcanti et al (1998)[138]determined the accuracy (validity) of 2D images reformatted from spiral CT for pre-surgical planning of dental implants in proximity to the mental foramen. The study was performed on eight cadaver heads (five males and three females), ages between 60 and 70 years. All specimens were edentulous posterior to the mental foramen. The heads were examined in a spiral CT scanner. High-resolution, 1 mm thick axial slices were obtained with 1 mm/sec table feed at 120 kVp and 150 mA. A low frequency filter cut-off was used in the reconstruction algorithm. Linear measurements were made by two oral radiologists independently from the superior border of the mental foramen to the crest of the alveolar process and from the inferior border of the mental foramen to the mandibular inferior border. The soft tissues were removed and physical measurements were made using a 3 Space (Polhemus, Colchester, VT) electromagnetic digitizer with a personal computer running Windows 95. The result were compared between the two sets of measurements made on the 2 DCT reconstructions and the physical measurements. The differences between the measurements were not statistically significant: for the distance between the alveolar crest and the superior border of the mental foramen (P=0.9) and for the inferior border of the mental foramen and the inferior border (P=0.7). Author concluded that spiral CT allowed a high degree of accuracy when planning dental implants in proximity to the mental foramen, making it possible to formulate a more accurate diagnosis and treatment plan.

Diniz et al (2008)[139]compared conventional radiograph with for implant placement for presurgical treatment planning of implant placement. 29 patients were selected, having 120 potential sites in 69 edentulous areas, out of that 7 implant sites excluded. Periapical, panoramic and cross-sectional tomographic radiographs were taken for all the patients. A Siemens Heliodent dental X-ray unit was used for periapical exams, with exposure values of 70 kV, 10mA and 0.16 -0.25 s, according to anatomic region. Panoramic and tomographic exams were undertaken using the Cranex Tome unit, with magnifying factor 1.5. The exposure values were 60-73 kV, 8-10 mA and 15 -19s for panoramic images, and 60-73 Kv, 1-6.4 mA and 46s for cross sectional images. Two independent experienced dental surgeons were invited to carry out pre-surgical treatment planning, considering 4 parameters like length and width of implants, need for bone grafting and need for other surgical procedures (bone augmentation, sinus lifting, nerve repositioning or distraction osteogenesis). Implant length and width was determined by using a transparent template with different implant sizes and appropriate magnification factor, superimposed upon the radiograph. Implant widths were scored from 1 to 3, corresponding to 7, 8.5, 10, 11.5, 13 and 15 mm lengths, respectively. Implant dimensions were limited by anatomical landmarks, such as an inferior alveolar canal, mental foramen, maxillary sinus, nasal cavity and incisive foramen. After clinical examination, pre-surgical planning was carried out in two stages: 1) using only periapical and panoramic images 2) after the first stage with the addition of the tomographic images. Implant length and width remained unchanged in 60.2% and 87.2% of cases respectively. No difference in length ($p = 0.576$) and width ($p = 1$) scores was observed in treatment planning with and without tomography. Variation in implant dimensions was not affected by location of edentulous areas. Bone grafting and other surgical procedures significantly changed after tomograms ($p < 0.001$), independent of the location of edentulous areas. In 15.8% and 5.3% of cases bone grafting and other procedures were planned only after tomograms, respectively. Significant difference were observed in all maxillary and mandibular regions. Author concluded that the use of conventional spiral as an adjuvant to conventional radiograph may help implant surgeons in pre-surgical treatment planning, especially when bone grafting and other surgical procedures were part of treatment plan.

Shahbazian et al (2010)[140]evaluated the maxillary sinus anatomy using spiral computed tomography in order to obtain more accurate information on the morphology, variation, volume and the amount of maxillary bone adjacent to the sinus. 101 consecutive patients with Maxillary sinus computed tomography

(CT) data were assessed. In which 30 patients (14 males, 16 females; aged 20 to 70 years; mean age = 53.8 years) were edentulous and 71 were partially edentulous (36 males, 35 females; aged 22 to 80 years; mean age = 52.8 years). Measurement of the patient's spiral CT scans employed with 1) The minimum and maximum alveolar bone height was measured on cross-sectional images between alveolar crest and maxillary sinus floor, as measured parallel to each tooth or scan prosthesis axis. 2)The size of the maxillary sinus according to anteroposterior (AP) and mediolateral (ML) diameters of the sinus was measured at 5, 10, 15 and 20 mm above the most apical level of the maxillary sinus floor and 3) Mucosal thickening of the maxillary sinus was defined as the existence of soft tissue structures thickness > 4 mm. The maxillary sinus was also assessed morphologically, by determining the anterior and posterior extends of the maxillary sinus, in relation to the respective teeth or estimated tooth sites. At the same time the occurrence of sinus septa was noted on axial and sagittal slices. The result indicated that the alveolar bone height was significantly higher in the premolar regions in comparison to the molar region (n =46. p< 0.01). The age showed negative relation to bone dimension (r= -0.32, p= 0.04). Anterior and posterior border of the maxillary sinuses were mostly located in the first premolar (49%) and second molar (84%) regions respectively. Maxillary sinus septa were identified in 47% of the maxillary antra. The present sample did not allow revealing any significant difference (p>0.05) in the maxillary sinus dimensions for partially dentate and edentulous subjects. Author concluded that cross-sectional imaging can be used in order to obtain more accurate information on the morphology, variation, and the amount of maxillary bone adjacent to the maxillary sinus.

Chen et al (2001)[141] used spiral dental CT in evaluating dental implantation. Twenty patients (age: 20~82 years with a mean of 51 years; 11 males and 9 females) were included in this study. They received the spiral dental CT examination for dental implantation. The transaxial jaw region tomograms produced a lateral topogram of the skull base. The scanning protocal on axial section was that the thickness of the section, 1 mm; table feed 1.5 mm; pitch, 1.5; rotation time, 1/s; filter kernel, AH 70 and at the voltage and the current of 120 kv and 90 mA, respectively. In order to position the dental implant, a line was projected either 1 parallel to the alveolar bone of the upper jaw or parallel to tooth bed of the lower jaw, or parallel to upper and lower occlusal planes of both jaws. A reconstruction of a 1 mm-thick image was reviewed. Then spiral dental software was used for reconstruction of the jaw, in addition to panoramic reconstruction. Axial scans reveal the exterior of the horizontal jaw bone, whereas panoramic scans show the width of bucco-lingual cavity, the height and width of the alveolar jaw bone. Teeth implantation was not indicated for the patients who wear removable dental prostheses for a long time or who have thin and narrow alveolar bone (<0.8 cm in thickness, < 0.4 cm in width). Author concluded that the development of spiral dental CT improved the quality of dental images. A precise preoperation evaluation will prevent injury to nerves and other important anatomical structures in maxillofacial region. The spiral dental CT method saved time in comparison with the conventional tomography.

Bou Serhal et al (2000)[32] evaluated the accuracy of the spiral tomographic technique to assess bone quantity for pre-operative implant planning in the posterior maxilla. Six dry human adult skulls edentulous in the maxillary sinus region were used in this study. Three sites were selected in the left posterior maxilla and marked with gutta percha meaning a total of 18 sites (6x3=18) for interpretation. Bone height and width were measured on the tomographs and after sectioning also on the skulls. The values obtained from the measurements on tomographs were divided by an enlargement factor of 1.5 (as defined by the manufacturer) and then compared with those from the real measurements on the skulls. The result showed that all tomographs were considered satisfactory for measurements. A slight difficulty to locate the floor of the sinus was noticed in some instances at the most distal site. The tomographs had a mean enlargement factor of 1.49 (SD 0.05) both for horizontal and vertical measurements. The mean difference between the corrected tomographic measurements (/1.5) and the real measurements was +0.24 mm (SD 0.19 mm) for both horizontal and vertical measurements. Those corrected measurements were found to be larger (overestimated) than the skull measurements in 33.3% of the cases. This difference was not statistically significant *($P<0.05$).* Author concluded that spiral tomography using the recently developed Cranex Tome reveals sufficient information and detail for pre-operative planning of a limited edentulous region.

Scanora units give considerably lower radiation doses than does CT and their cost is approximately one-fifth of that of a CT machine (Tammisalo et al 1992).[136] Nevertheless, when performing the multiple tomographic cuts needed for imaging an entire maxillary bone, the total dosage is higher than that for a reformatted CT scan examination (Kassebaum et al 1992).[142] In complex situations where multiple implants are to be placed throughout the arch of the jaw, conventional X-ray tomography becomes impractical, as it is extremely time-consuming to produce a large number of cross-sectional tomograms (Schwarz et al 1990).[48]

F. LINEAR TOMOGRAPHY :

Cross-sectional tomographic X-ray machines produce images of slices or layers (focal plane) of the body by using the movement of the X-ray beam and film (connected by a fulcrum bar) during an exposure to blur unwanted body parts. Linear tomographic motion is one-dimensional and produces blurring of adjacent sections in one dimension. Complex (multi-directional) tomographic motion—circular, elliptical, spiral and hypocycloidal tomography-is obtained by using the 2-dimensional movement of the tube and film and produces relatively uniform blurring of the patient's anatomy adjacent to the tomographic plane.

Cross-sectional tomography has been successfully applied in dental implant radiography (Eckerdal et al 1986).[143] Cross-sectional tomographs have been shown to be more precise than panoramic radiographs when measuring the distance between the alveolar crest and the mandibular canal (Lindh et al 1989).[94] Several studies have shown that tomographic images of the posterior mandible allow better visualization of the mandibular canal than the other available radiographic techniques (Klinge B 1989, Lindh C and Petersson 1989).[106,94]

Rockenbach et al (2003)[144]compared linear tomography measurement with panoramic radiograph for evaluation of mandibular implant sites. Twenty dry edentulous hemimandibles were selected in this study with 1.5 cm distal from the anterior limit of the mental foramen. A metallic wire was fixed at the buccal portion of the alveolar ridge, serving as reference in the radiographic exams for the localization of the proposed research area. The examinations were made utilizing the Vera View Scope X–600 equipment, in which each mandible specimen was positioned with its base parallel to the ground and with the median line coinciding with the luminous indicator of the equipment. Mandibles were fixed firmly to the chin support utilizing a block of wax to avoid any movement during radiography. Initially, a panoramic radiograph was taken and, through the scale present in this radiograph, the area for the linear tomography was identified. In cases in which the metallic wire was located in an intermediate position, a more mesial area was chosen. Three tomographic slices (5.0 mm thick) were obtained in each selected region. Four measurements were made. The images obtained were drawn on acetate paper and the hemimandibles cut at the demarcated area.

The measurements were made using a digital electronic pachymeter. The values found for the radiographic images were compared to those obtained in the mandibular specimens and submitted to statistical evaluation by the Wilcoxon test. Author concluded that the linear tomography overestimated the measurements obtained in the mandibular specimens, whereas the panoramic radiography presented values close to the true measurements of the dry mandibles.

Todd et al (1993)[145] evaluated the diagnostic interpretation of tomographic images by individual dental implant team members, and compared the precision of Linear tomography (LT) measurements with the corresponding CT cross-sectional images. Five partially edentulous human cadaver mandibles with intact periodontium were obtained for tomographic evaluation. Edentulous areas were then selected as the proposed implant. The position of the implant sites was identified in the Stents by condensing warmed gutta-percha into holes prepared with a 2-mm twist drill. Each mandible with its stent in place was then radiographed using both CT and LT. Tomogram tracings were compared to each other and to the equivalent CT cross-sectional image to determine the precision of the measurements. One mandible was sectioned to verify the accuracy of the CT images. Repeated measures analysis of variance of the measurements made from the LT and CT scans showed significant statistical differences between team members. Multiple cross sectional views facilitated identification of the inferior alveolar canal in the majority of CT scans, whereas image blurring inherent to LT resulted in the inability of team members to identify the canal in 14% to 50% of the images. Volume averaging within the CT slice aperture was found capable of producing a magnification error of short dense objects. CT and LT must both be interpreted cautiously because of innate technique pecularities that can lead to measurement errors. Author conclude that the wide variation in interpretation of the linear tomograms and frequent inability to identify the inferior alveolar canal made this technique less valuable than the reformatted CT when planning dental surgical procedures.

The disadvantages of using conventional linear tomograms is the lack of adequate cross-referencing with standard lateral, frontal, and panoramic radiographs (Schwarz et al 1989).[146] Thus, a mental transformation is required prior to, and during, surgery. Teeth, particularly those with large metallic restorations adjacent to the area of interest, may obscure the tomographic image. Another disadvantage is limited resolution caused by use of an intensifying screen cassette, making the identification of anatomical structures and assessment of bone topography more difficult (Todd et al 1993).[145]

Tomographic images are always magnified because of the relationships between focus-film and film-object distances. Since all the structures in the tomographic plane are at the same distance between focus and film, the tomographic images are free from distortion. They have a uniform magnification and the magnification factor depends on the relationship between the focus-film and film-object distances. Multi-directional tomography provides images superior in quality to linear tomography because of more uniform blurring (Grondahl et al 1991, Tammisalo et al 1992).[147,136]

G. TRANSTOMOGRAPHY/ SECTIONAL TOMOGRAPHY :

It has been reported that the use of transtomography for the placement of implants using a radiopaque radiographic guide can provide the necessary and accurate information for implant placement. Modern tomograms can give good accuracy, but care has to be taken in interpretation of the images (Peltola JS 2004).[148] Blurring has been noted in the posterior maxilla, due to overlying bony structures and posterior mandible (Bolin A et al 1996).[31] This technique enables the appreciation of spatial relationship between the critical structures and the implant site and quantification of the geometry of the implant site. The tomographic layers are thick and have adjacent structures that are blurred and superimposed on the image, limiting the usefulness of this technique for individual sites, especially in the anterior regions where the geometry of the alveolus changes rapidly. This technique is not useful for determining the differences in most bone densities or identifying disease at the implant site (Monsour PA 2008, Schwarz et al 1989).[20,146]

Bousquet (2007)[149]evaluated accuracy of transtomography for the placement of implants using a radiopaque radiographic guide. 9 partially edentulous patients (six female and three male patients), age ranging from 31 years to 76 years (mean age 53 years), were included in this study. The implants were inserted in 11 sites (1 incisor site in the maxilla; 7 molar and 3 premolar sites in the mandible). All patients were examined using a ProMax panoramic unit implemented with transtomographic Technique. This digital panoramic unit can create image layer thickness ranging from 1 mm to 36 mm and combines a longitudinal and cross-sectional transtomogram in one composite image. An image layer thickness of 3 mm was chosen for this study. The exposure values were 66 kV, 1 mA and 8 s. Implant position and length were estimated by measuring the crestal width and the distance from the top of the ridge to the critical anatomic structures. At each implant site, cross-sectional and longitudinal intraoperative transtomograms were taken through a radiopaque reference guide to control and adjust the drilling axis. The effective axis on post-operative transtomograms was compared with the planned axis correction estimated on intraoperative images. Radiopaque guides, used as the gold standard, were measured on intraoperative cross-sectional slices to evaluate image distortion. Comparison of the pre-operative, intraoperative and postoperative transtomograms showed no artefact produced by either the titanium guide or the dental implant. In 7 sites (63.6%) out of 11 sites, the crest width was less than 7 mm (ranging from 5.2 mm to 6.5 mm) and a lingual undercut or a buccal concavity was obvious on pre-operative tomograms in 8 sites (72.7%) out of 11 sites. All intraoperative transtomograms gave clear images of the cortical plates and information of drilling length and axis which allowed the surgeon to adjust pilot drilling axis in 6 sites (54.5%) out of 11 sites, including sites with narrow bone ridges. The effective axis of the implant on the post-operative transtomogram, compared with the estimated axis rectification planned when necessary on the intraoperative transtomography, showed an angle difference ranging from 0.88 to 3.48. The image distortion on cross-sectional slices ranged from0.03 mm to 0.52 mm, resulting in a distortion ratio ranging from0%to 6%when expressed in percentages. Author concluded that transtomographic examination performed with a radiographic reference guide during implant surgery can provide the necessary and accurate information for implant placement.

Peltola and Mattila (2004)[148] evaluated the accuracy and ability of four different panoramic radiography units to produce cross-sectional images of the posterior mandible using microradiographs as a gold standard. Cross-sectional tomograms were obtained from a human cadaver mandible using four panoramic radiography units, capable of producing cross-sectional images. Cross sectional tomographs were taken from two edentulous and one dentate area (mandibular right first and second molar and mandibular left second premolar area) and marked by gluing an orthodontic tube onto the alveolar crest. A second tube was glued on the buccal aspect of the mandible on a line drawn from the first tube perpendicular to the inferior border of the mandible. The marks were used to verify the correct sites for tomography and the position of the mandible. The mandible was fastened on a tripod stand with the inferior border horizontal to assist positioning in the

X-ray unit. Four different linear distances were measured from each radiograph. The mandible was then cut into 4 mm thick slices at three marked places. These slices were microradiographed and used as the gold standard for measurements made from each cross-sectional tomogram. Of all measurements only the thickness of the mandible in the radiographs taken with the OP-100 differed significantly (P, 0.021) from the gold standard. In the interexaminer variation, the agreement was 85% and Kappa index 0.68. In the intraexaminer reproducibility, the agreement was 76.7% and Kappa indices 0.52 and 0.50. Author concluded that All X-ray units studied provided acceptable results in edentulous areas for implant site assessment in this limited examination. Interexaminer and intraexaminer variations can be large, but measurement accuracy can be improved by making several measurements to calculate the mean value.

Welander et al (2004)[150] described how advanced panoramic machines that combine a translational movement with a pendular movement of the beam and detector make direct digital transtomographic images and can be utilized for the same purposes as conventional tomography. Transtomography produces almost instant results and allows quick measurements on the screen with a computed program. This made transtomography more appropriate than conventional tomography using films or PSP plates. In addition, the panoramic machine's compact size allowed it to be installed in the operating room. The surgeon rapidly and conveniently performed intraoperative investigations in the shortest time (with no discomfort to the patient) as the panoramic machine was within a few paces of the operating table.

With a radiographic guide and transtomography, the risks of critical anatomic zones injury and of cortical plate perforation were minimized, allowing implant placement in all cases, including sites presenting a narrow ridge, a buccal concavity or a lingual undercut. The tomographic layers are thick and have adjacent structures that are blurred and superimposed on the image, limiting the usefulness of this technique for individual sites, especially in the anterior regions where the geometry of the alveolus changes rapidly. This technique is not useful for determining the differences in most bone densities or identifying disease at the implant site (Monsour and Dudhia 2008, Welander et al 2004).[20,150]

H. INTERACTIVE COMPUTED TOMOGRAPHY:

One of the most significant advances in CT is interactive computed tomography (ICT), which addresses many of the limitations of CT (Moreira CR et al 2009, Jacobs R 2002) This technique was developed to bridge the gap in information transfer between the radiologist and the practitioner. This technique enables the radiologist to transfer the imaging study to the practitioner as a computer file and enables the practitioner to view and interact with the imaging study on a personal computer. The dentist's computer becomes a diagnostic radiologic workstation, with tools to measure the length and the width of the alveolus, measure bone quality and change the window and level of the grayscale of the study to enhance the perception of critical structures (Engelman 1988).[19]

An important feature of ICT is that the dentist and radiologist can perform electronic surgery (ES) by selecting and placing arbitrary-sized cylinders that simulate root form implants in the images. With an appropriately designed diagnostic template, ES can be performed to develop the patient's treatment plan electronically in 3D. Superimnosed on the CBCT image, electronic implants can be virtually previewed at arbitrary positions and orientations with respect to each other, the alveolus, critical structures and the prospective occlusion and esthetics. ES and ICT enable the development of a 3D treatment plan that is integrated with the patient's anatomy and can be visualized before surgery (Dreiseidler T et al 2009, Chau AC 2009).[151,152]

Moussa et al (2015)[153] evaluated the dental implant surface roughness by a computerized tomographic data analysis system. 9 completely edentulous patients were rehabilitated by conventional maxillary complete denture and mandibular implant retained over denture in which two implant systems with different surface roughness produced by blasting the surface with resorbable particles of tri-calcium phosphate were used. A total of 18 implants were inserted in the mandibular anterior region. Implants were allocated randomly to the right or left sides of the mandible. Peri implant bone density in Hounsfield Units (HU) was evaluated by Computerized Tomographic (CT) images to judge the behavior of an implant system under functional loading, where DICOM raw data was imported into the analysis proposed system to correlate the bone density regarding to the HU values. Images were magnified and implant surface was divided into three vertical regions: Coronal (C), Middle (M) and Apical (A) on each axial surface of the implant (Buccal, Lingual, Mesial and Distal) .Bone density was measured in rectangular areas in all three zones along all implant surfaces; buccal and lingual surfaces in the sagittal plane, and on mesial and distal surfaces in the coronal plane. Bone density in the selected regions was displayed automatically through the software program used, in terms of mean value and standard deviation of HU. The examiner measured the bone density of each region three times on three successive slices through the center of each implant and in a plane anterior and a plane posterior to the central plane. The mean peri-implant bone density value at the coronal zone of buccal, lingual, mesial, and distal surfaces of the two implants, was calculated at 0, 3, and 6 months and compared with the corresponding values of the middle and apical zones. The average of such a density profile represents a line integral, which was an indicator for the degree of osseointegration. Results was compared with clinical readings and previous findings, which showed difference in peri implant bone density around regularly patterned and randomly patterned implant surfaces. Therefore, author concluded that Bone density monitoring was a useful diagnostic tool to judge the behavior of an implant system under functional loading.

Geng et al (2015)[154] evaluated the clinical outcomes of implants placed using different types of CAD/CAM surgical guides, including partially guided and totally guided templates, and determined the accuracy of the different guides. 24 patients (13 men and 11 women; mean age, 41.6 ± 15.2 years; range, 25-65 years) with missing teeth or edentulous jaws were included in this study. In total, 111 implants were placed using CAD/CAM surgical guides. After implant insertion, the positions and angulations of the placed implants relative to those of the planned ones were determined using special software that matched pre- and postoperative computed tomography (CT) images, and deviations were calculated and compared between the different guides and templates. The mean angular deviations were 1.72 and 2.71, the mean deviations in position at the neck were 0.27 and 0.69 mm, the mean deviations in position at the apex were 0.37 and 0.94 mm, and the mean depth deviations were 0.32 and 0.51mm with tooth- and mucosa-supported stereolithographic guides, respectively ($P < .05$ for all). The mean distance deviations when partially guided (29 implants) and totally guided templates (30 implants) were 0.54 mm and 0.89 mm, respectively, at the neck and 1.10 mm and 0.81 mm, respectively, at the apex, with corresponding mean angular deviations of 2.56 and 2.90 ($P > .05$ for all).Author concluded that CAD/CAM surgical guides can improve the precision of dental implant placement.

Moustafa et al (2012)[155]generated a new interactive 3-D model based on the radiological information offered by medium-dose CT technology for use in 3-D analyses including functional imaging and real time imaging for guiding interventional procedures and compared with quality of 3-D model retrieved from CBCT imaging and also meshing of the 3-D model from the CT scan to help on simulation of occlusal loads on dental im-plants. Nine completely edentulous male patients were scheduled for prosthetic rehabilitation by con-ventional maxillary complete denture and mandibular over denture retained by two dental implants. One patient 63 of years old, was selected for a pilot study after his approval. Clinical estimation of bucco-lingual width of the lower edentulous ridge was done by Boley's gauge and the overlying soft tissue thickness by sharpened periodontal probe after employment of local an-aesthesia. The patient was then referred for radiographic examination by 3-D CT (GE MEDICAL SYSTEMS/BrightSpeed S) with DICOM format output and after one month and before implant placement he was imaged by CBCT (Planmeca ProMax® TDV320077) with DAP format. For generating a 3-D model, 3-D visualization was per-formed by means of triangulation of a segmented 3-D area. The number of triangles determines the quality of the re-construction: the more triangles, the higher the quality. Two methods for reducing the number of triangles was used, Image matrix reduction and triangle reduction. In this study an interactive 3-D model was retrieved from Computed Tomography (CT) images utilizing, a proposed software was used to obtain high image quality of the jaw bones scanned by 3-D CT compared with Cone Beam Computed tomography (CBCT) output. Identification of different anatomical regions set for mandible cortical and spongy bones with soft tissues by generated 3-D models and validated with real measurements from solid model. Author concluded that it helped at diagnosis and pre-surgical process and provides a direct meshing lossless method for the FEA to ensure that all nu-merical analysis that can be determined from these models gain the reality and be more accurate than other classical methods.

Yatzkair (2014)[156] analyzed accuracy of computer-guided dental implantation using a human cadaver model with reduced experimental variability. Twenty-eight (28) dental implants representing 12 clinical cases were placed in four cadaver heads using a static guided implantation template. An impression of both jaws was taken, and a cast was made. A specific CT guide with facial markers was created and used for pre-implantation scans of each cadaver head. The CT scan was used with a specific setup to obtain the CBCT radiographic scans, which allowed for scanning the heads before and after implantation without altering alignment. After implantation, CBCT scans were retaken. Measurements between the location of implants in CT at the time of planning and after implantation were made at the coronal and apical levels to determine the distance between the implant and buccal and lingual bone, and adjacent (mesial) implant/teeth. No significant differences were seen between planned and implanted measurements. Average deviation of an implant from its planning radiograph was 0.8 mm, which was within the range of variability expected from CT analysis. Therefore, author concluded that implant planning with 3D and guided templates should include a safety distance of 1 mm and also suggested that guided implantation can be used safely in difficult cases near anatomic structures.

The evolution in hardware has been followed by refinements of software allowing 3-dimensional computer-assisted tomography-based implant planning. Interactive computer software programs now allow reformatted CT data to be analyzed on a personal computer when developing a treatment plan.

The 3-dimensional CT planning system is a reliable tool for the preoperative assessment of potential implant sites. A recently developed interactive 3-dimensional CT software program (SimPlant; Materialse, Leuven, Belgium) has made it possible to visualize the anatomical structures in a 3-dimensional mode on computer monitors for interactive implant placement. SimPlant uses raw data (DICOM files) from the CT scan to display reformatted CT images for the inspection of the bony anatomy of the alveolar ridges. Bone height and width can be easily measured from point to point. The planned implant length and diameter can therefore be determined. The angulation of the planned implant can be adjusted for optimal orientation with respect to the natural teeth and bony anatomy. The esthetic and biomechanical considerations (implant alignment) are made easier with 3-dimensional images (Verstreken K et al 1998).[157] These interactive, reformatted cross-sectional images, used together with 3-dimensional reconstruction planning, give a better prognostic value than conventional reformatted cross-sectional CT planning for implant lengths (Jacobs R 1998).[47]

The CT scan data obtained from the SimPlant software can be used to produce sterolithographic models for 3- dimensional visualization for planning complex maxillofacial surgery. There are two techniques available for making sterolithographic models (Lambrecht JT et al 1995).[158] The first technique applies laser technology in which a sterolithographic model is built up, layer by layer, with resin solution. A resin layer is solidified when its surface is struck with the laser. Another technique uses a computer-aided milling machine. Surgical guides, and provisional and permanent restorations for implants, can all be fabricated using sterolithographic models (Sudbrink SD 2005).[159]At this time ICT is the most accurate imaging technique for implant imaging and surgery but suffers some limitations. ES enables placement of electronic implants in the imaging study but the refinement and exact relative orientation of the implant positions is difficult and cumbersome (Petrikowski CG et al 1989).[160]

CHAPTER 6:
IMAGING STENTS

When placing dental implants, a flap is traditionally elevated to better visualize the implant recipient sites and flap elevation also provides that some anatomical landmarks (i.e., foramina, maxillary sinuses), are clearly identified and protected. To minimize the possibility of post-operative peri-implant tissue loss and to overcome the challenge of soft tissue management during or after surgery, the concept of flapless implant surgery has been introduced for the patients with the sufficient bone volume in the implant recipient site (Campelo and Camara 2002, Rocci et al 2003).[161,162] However, when deciding whether to place dental implants without raising a flap, several considerations should be kept in mind. To minimize the risk of perforation and incorrect implant alignment, computed tomography (CT)-guided surgical stents can be used to help the dental practitioner to give the implant the proper axial direction. To calculate the "true" size distortion in a certain area of a radiograph, it has been suggested to use a metal marker of known dimensions as a reference, which is included in the radiograph close to the area of interest (Jacobs 1998).[47] Several other methods have been suggested in the literature for calibration purposes (Borrow et al 1996),[163] e.g., the use of cylindrical metal markers or Gutta Percha markers.

Cassetta et al (2013)[164] analyzed immediate loading in complete edentulous patients, using a dedicated software that provides beforehand both the information for a guided implant placement and the creation of a temporary prosthesis. A 45 years old male completely edentulous, required a fixed implant-supported prosthetic rehabilitation was treated. The patient underwent a CT-Dentascan wearing a “scan prosthesis”. CT data were imported in the software to plan the exact position of the implants. Following these guidelines a mucosa-supported surgical template was developed. A flapless implant site preparation was performed. 22 implants were placed in a complete edentulous patient. The abutments were positioned and the impressions for the final restoration were taken. The patient received immediately the temporary prosthesis that was prepared prior to the surgery in the dental laboratory. Due to the flapless surgery, post-operative swelling and pain was limited. The computer-aided planning and the template guided surgery allowed to place a temporary fixed prosthesis within hours and an aesthetic and functional final restoration within some days. Therefore, author concluded that the described procedure proved to be really effective, allowing to face, in a single time, surgical and prosthetic phases and allowing to deliver the prosthesis to the patient immediately after the implant insertion.

Schropp et al (2009)[165] evaluated the impact of a reference metal ball for calibration of periapical and panoramic radiographs on the preoperative selection of implant size for three implant systems. 70 patients (45 female, 25 male) with single tooth implants were included in this study. Presurgical radiographs (70 panoramic and 43 periapical) of 70 single implant sites were evaluated by three observers (one radiologist, one surgeon, and one prosthodontist) with the intent to select the appropriate implant size. Four reference marks corresponding to the margins of the metal ball were manually placed on the digital image by means of computer software. Additionally, an implant with proper dimensions for the respective site was outlined by manually placing four reference marks. The diameter of the metal ball and the unadjusted length and width of the implant were calculated. Implant size was adjusted according to a “standard” calibration method (SCM; magnification factor 1.25 in panoramic images and 1.05 in periapical images) and according to a reference ball calibration method (RCM; true magnification). For the periapical radiographs, a different implant size was selected in at least 40% of the cases when comparing the values obtained with SCM to the unadjusted ones and in at least 56% of the cases when comparing the values from RCM with the unadjusted ones. When comparing SCM with RCM, there was a change in implant size in 24% of the cases. For the panoramic radiographs, when comparing the values obtained with SCM with those from RCM, a different implant size was selected in at least 46% of the cases. Implant size changes between SCM and RCM in panoramic radiographs were more pronounced in the maxillary anterior region (62%) than in the premolar (41%) and molar (38%) regions and more in the mandibular premolar region (41%) than in the molar region (24%). Therefore, author concluded that The use of a reference metal ball for calibration of periapical and panoramic radiographs during treatment planning seems advantageous since it allowed a more precise selection of the implant size.

Ozan et al (2007)[166] evaluated the implant survival of early loaded implants placed using flapless or conventional flapped protocols and determined the bone density of implant recipient sites using computerized tomography-guided surgical stents. A total of 12 patients (seven females, five males), mean age 46 ±9 treated with 59 implants were included in this study. Existing edentulous spans were allocated into four groups; anterior mandible, posterior mandible, anterior maxilla and posterior maxilla. There were eight anterior mandibular sites, 17 posterior mandibular sites, 16 anterior maxillary sites and 18 posterior maxillary sites. The implants used in this study included 59 Tapered SwissPlus implants with diameters of 3.7 mm, 4.1 mm, 4.8 mm and lengths of 8 mm, 10 mm, 12 mm. A spiral model CT machine† were utilized for the preoperative evaluation of the jaw bones for each patient. 3-D STENTCAD software was used for determining the locations and directions of implants placement. The mean bone density of each implant area has been measured using the STENTCAD software on sagital CT images. The mean bone density value of each implant recipient site was recorded in Hounsfield units (HU). All implants were placed using CT guided surgical stents. The early loading protocols included 2 months of healing in the mandible and 3 months of healing in the maxilla. Single-implant crowns, implant-supported fixed partial dentures, and implant-retained over dentures were delivered to the patients. Of 59 implants placed, one was lost in the conventional flapped group within the first month of healing, meaning overall implant survival rate of 98.3% average 9 months later. The highest average bone density value (801 ± 239 HU) was found in the anterior mandible, followed by 673 ± 449 HU for the posterior maxilla, 669 ± 346 HU for the anterior maxilla and 538± 271 HU for the posterior mandible. Therefore, author concluded that flapless surgical approach using CT-guided surgical stents may be a feasible option for implant placement.

Presurgical imaging can be enhanced by use of an imaging stent that helps relate radiographic image & its information to a precise anatomic location or potential surgical site. The implant sites can be identified by radiographic spheres or rods retained within acrylic stent. These can subsequently be used as a surgical guide to orient the insertion angle of the guide bar & ultimately the angle of implant. Since the metallic markers produce artifacts in CT, only non metallic radio-opaque markers, eg .guttapercha, resins, composites are to be used.

CHAPTER 7

IMAGING SOFTWARES

The computer software uses the radiopaque markers which have been placed in the scanning denture, to perform an accurate fusion of the two separate scans. Resulting from this fusion is an exact representation of the patient's bone structure and scanning denture in 3D space. At this point, the virtual surgical procedure can be performed. In 1986, Fellingham et al first demonstrated the use of interactive graphics and 3D modelling for surgical planning, prosthesis, and implant design. By using the software, the dental team can select implants of specific lengths and diameters from a database of most commercially available implants and it can reproduce a 3D replica of exact dimensions in the desired location on the computer model of the patient's jaw. This 3D planning software allows an undistorted visualisation of the jawbone in four views: axial, cross-sectional, panoramic and 3D reformatted data. It allows 3D visualisation of all the anatomical structures which are situated within the bone and the prosthesis. Following is a flow chart which shows procedure which is followed once the data is obtained:

Once the computer simulation is completed

It is saved as a "sim'' file which is sent to the processing centre via e-mail

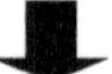

This file transfers geometrical information which consists of numerous triangles.

This triangulated data is the interface to the stereolithographic apparatus (SLA) (Lal et al 2006)[167]

The software is available for both computed tomography (SURRLAN) and reformatted computed tomography (Denta Scan, SimPlant). Other softwares like Procera Software (Nobelbiocare, Sweden, Vimplant (CyberMed, Seoul, Korea) are also available. These programs provide an interactive platform permitting analysis of potential implant sites for bone quantity, quality and morphology (Shetty and Benson 1999, Gray et al 1996).[44,168] SIMPLANT software has provided the doctor with the capability to interact with CT scan data on a personal computer, allowing for pre-operative simulation of implant placement, prosthetic simulation and bone augmentation simulation that makes SIMPLANT the state-of-the-art imaging tool for dental implants. With the use of interactive CT, not only is the surgical phase of treatment planned, but the prosthetic phase is planned as well.

Zhao et al (2014)[169] used 3D implant planning software combined with a laser scanning technique to manufacture surgical templates with a computed aided design design / computed aided manufacturing (CAD/ CAM) technique and evaluated it's precision in clinical cases. A total of 11 partially edentulous patients with four men (35 to 72 years, mean 48 years) and seven women (31 to 62 years, mean 42.9 years) were included in this study. Cone beam computed tomography (CBCT) was applied to each patient using an E-WOO machine (DCTPRO-46; Vatech).

The scanning conditions were 90 kV, 10 mA, and 24 S (metal artifacts reduction condition). The upper margin of the area to be scanned was the line connecting the bilateral tragus. The lower margin was the inferior margin of the mandibular bone. 3D configurations of the restored diagnostic casts were subsequently recorded by a 3D laser scanner (3D Scanner Opticscan-DM; Shining 3D Tech), which then presented the information about each patient's mucosa and dentition. 3D laser scanning data were also imported into Simplant software and were matched with the a foresaid CT data into a single coordinate system with the aid of an image spatial registration technique. Implant positions were planned in the software with a computer-aided design technique, and surgical templates were fabricated with a rapid prototyping technique. These templates were used to guide implant placement surgery. The mean value of linear deviation was 1.00 mm (range 0 to 2.16 mm) for implant shoulder and 1.26 mm (range 0.51 to 2.86 mm) for the implant apex. The mean angular deviation was 4.74 degress (0.37 to 10.28 degrees). Deviations were higher in the posterior regionthan anterior. The tooth-supported template provided higher precision than did the tooth/mucosa-supported template, but no statistically significant difference was found. Author concluded that Computer-guided implant surgery with a CAD/CAM technique provided dentists a good platform for preoperative planning, precise implant insertion, and ideal rehabilitation.

`Ruppin et al (2008)[170] Evaluated of the accuracy of three different computer-aided surgery systems in dental implantology. 20 human cadaver mandibles were used in this vitro study. The mandibles were mounted on acrylic plates to allow anatomically correct and fully reproducible positioning in the CT. Steel spheres with a diameter of 1mm were attached to the bone and the acrylic plate to serve as fiducialmarkers for matching the two CT data sets (pre- and postoperative). The mandibles were subjected to a high resolution multislice CT scan. The mandibles were divided into three groups. Forty implants were planned in each group. Planning was performed using the SimPlant One Shott software in the first, the RoboDent LapDoc Accedos software in the second and the Artma Virtual Patient software in the third group. Implant placement was performed using either optical tracking or stereolithographic splints. Postoperative CT scans were used to obtain the achieved implant positions. A semi-automatic approach was developed to compare planned and achieved implant positions. Deviations between planned and achieved positions were measured for each implant in position (▲ xy), depth (▲ z) and axis (▲ ϕ). In the first group using the SimPlant/ SurgiGuidet splint system, the total application errors between planned and achieved implant position were 1.5 mm for start point deviation ▲xy, 0.6 mm for insertion depth deviation ▲ z and 7.9 for axis deviation ▲ ϕ . In the second group, using the RoboDent LapDoc Accedos tracking system, the total application errors between planned and achieved Implant position were 1 mm for start point deviation ▲xy, 0.6 mm for insertion depth deviation▲ z and 8.1 for axis deviation ▲ ϕ. In the third group, using the Artma Virtual Patientt tracking system, the total application errors between planned and achieved Implant position were 1.2 mm for start point deviation ▲xy, 0.8 mm for insertion depth deviation ▲z and 8.1 for axis deviation ▲ ϕ. No statistically significant differences were found between the three groups. Author concluded that despite the different techniques of transfer, no statistically significant differences were found between all groups. The accuracy achieved corresponded well with the spatial resolution of the CT Scans used.

Geng et al (2015)[154] evaluated the clinical outcomes of implants placed using different types of CAD/CAM surgical guides, including partially guided and totally guided templates, and determined the accuracy of the different guides. 24 patients (13 men and 11 women) with missing teeth or edentulous jaws requiring 111 implant placement were included in this study. After implant insertion, the positions and angulations of the placed implants relative to those of the planned ones were determined using special software that matched pre- and postoperative computed tomography (CT) images, and deviations were calculated and compared between the different guides and templates. Results: The mean angular deviations were 1.72 mm and 2.71mm, the mean deviations in position at the neck were 0.27mm and 0.69 mm, the mean deviations in position at the apex were 0.37 and 0.94 mm, and the mean depth deviations were 0.32 mm and 0.51 mm with tooth- and mucosa-supported stereolithographic guides, respectively ($P < .05$ for all). The mean distance deviations when partially guided (29 implants) and totally guided templates (30 implants) were used were 0.54 mm and 0.89 mm, respectively, at the neck and 1.10 ± 0.85 mm and 0.81 mm, respectively, at the apex, with corresponding mean angular deviations of 2.56° and 2.90°.Author concluded that CAD/CAM surgical guides can improve the precision of dental implant placement. Tooth-supported surgical guides may be more accurate than mucosa-supported guides, while partially guided templates can provide the same outcomes as totally guided templates, thus simplifying the surgical procedure.

Fortin et al (2001)[171]evaluatedthe Precision of transfer of preoperative planning for oral implants based on cone-beam CT-scan images through a robotic drilling machine. Three edentulous models were used for study purpose. The dry mandible was edentulous in both posterior regions, the plaster cast had a single missing incisor and was edentulous in both posterior regions and the dry maxilla had several single missing teeth. Several titanium tubes, of 2mm internal diameter and 10mm long, were inserted into the Master model (MM). Image-guided systems for oral implant placement consist of a software program for virtual implant placement and a position measurement system, which determines the spatial orientation and position of a drill to transfer the planned position onto a template or directly to the operating theater. In the Cad-ImplantA protocol (Praxim, Grenoble, France) (Fortin et al. 2000), the position measurement system was the Cad-Implant drilling machine, whose configuration can be tuned with 4 degrees of freedom because an axis in space has 4 degrees of freedom. To drill the template at the exact location, it was of primary importance to find a rigid mathematical transformation (T) between the RCS of the software program for virtual implant placement and the RCS of the drilling machine. Therefore, a mechanical device was built to make an acrylic resin cube including two tubes made of titanium in a very precise position, perpendicular and uncrossed. To determine the accuracy of the system, the ability of a 1.8-mm diameter drill to enter a 2.0-mm diameter, 10-mm-long titanium tube was inserted on the model with no contact. The drill entered the tubes with no contact and went beyond the end of the tube, the transfer error was less than 0.2 mm for translation and less than 1.1a for rotation. The method presented here is of low cost and high precision compared to other technological solutions such as tracking. Author concluded that further assessment in the surgical field should lead to daily use of this system for flapless surgery, to prepare a prosthesis prior to surgery for immediate loading, to reduce risk of injuring critical anatomical structures and to eliminate manual placement error.

Wanschitzet al (2002)[172] evaluated effectiveness of Computer-enhanced stereoscopic vision in a head-mounted display (HMD) for oral implant surgery. The HMD was equipped with two miniature computer monitors that project computer-generated graphics stereoscopically into the optical path. Its position was tracked by the navigation system's optical tracker and target structures was displayed in their true position over the operation site. In order to test this system's accuracy and spatial perception of the viewer, five interforaminal implants in three dry human mandibles were planned with visit and executed using the stereoscopic projection through the HMD. The deviation between planned and achieved position of the implants was measured on corresponding computed tomography (CT) scan images recorded postoperatively. The deviation between planned and achieved implant position at the jaw crest was 0.57 mm measured from the lingual, and 0.58 mm measured from the buccal cortex. At the tip of the implants the deviation was 0.77 mm at the lingual and 0.79 mm at the buccal cortex. The mean angular deviation between planned and executed implant position was 3.55 degrees. The study indicates that the concept of preoperative planning and transfer to the operative field by an HMD allows to achieve an average precision within 1 mm (range up to 3 mm) of the implant position and within 3 ^{0} deviation for the implant inclination (range up to 10^{0}). Author concluded that control during the drilling procedure was significantly improved by stereoscopic vision through the HMD resulting in a more accurate inclination of the implants.

Until the late 1980s, conventional radiographic techniques were considered as an acceptable standard for preoperative assessment and planning of dental implant patients. However, in present times, most diagnostic aids, such as, periapical and panoramic radiography or mounted study models are unable to provide complete comprehension of the dental arch anatomy. A surgical guide fabricated on a diagnostic study cast is endowed with unsatisfactory knowledge of the underlying anatomy. Moreover, the limitations of the conventional dental radiography, particularly, insufficient dimensional accuracy (magnification error, distortion error, setting error and position artefactsand inability to visualize anatomical structures in para-sagittal sections, further hinder accurate evaluation and result in unpredictable clinical outcomes. Thus, the limitations of the current clinical techniques often do not allow fabrication of surgical guides that are capable of accurately transferring planned implant placement intraoperatively (Lal et al 2006).[167] The present use of CAD/CAM processed surgical guides has provided a high degree of simplicity in morphologic diagnosis, determining the surgical procedure, and establishing the subsequent prognosis. Moreover, CAD/ CAM technology has facilitated flapless surgeries by improvising on pre-surgical planning. They have also facilitated restoration-driven surgeries by integrating.

The imaging modalities range from two dimensional projections to complex three dimensional imaging. The two dimensional modalities like conventional radiography are readily available, cost effective with least radiation exposure, but have limitations of magnifications and superimpositions. Therefore, in complex cases, more extensive and advanced radiographic evaluation is needed. Hence, cross-sectional imaging is increasingly considered essential for optimal implant placement and pre- and postoperative evaluation of the implant patient especially for complex reconstructions of edentulous ridges with multiple implants placement.

BIBLIOGRAPHY:

1. Turkyilmaz I, McGlumphy EA. Is there a lower threshold value of bone density for early loading protocols of dental implants?.J Oral Rehabil 2008; 35: 775–81.
2. Resnik, RR, Kircos L and Misch CE. Diagnostic Imaging and Techniques. Contemp Clin Dent.2008:38-67.
3. Benson BW and Shetty V. Dental Implants, In: Oral Radiology Principles and Interpretation, S.C. White & M. J. Pharoah 2009: 597-612.
4. Bragger U. Digital imaging in periodontal radiography. A review. J Clin Periodontol 1988; 15:551-57.
5. Webber RL, Ruttimann UE, Grondahl HG. X-ray image subtraction as a basis for assessment of periodontal changes. J Perio Res 1982; 17:509-11.
6. Matteson SR, Deahl ST. Advanced imaging methods. Crit Rev Oral Biol Med 1996; 7:346-95.
7. Grondahl K, Kullendorff B. Detectability of artificial marginal bone lesions as a function of lesion depth. J Clin Periodontol 1988; 15:156-62.
8. Christgau M, Hiller KA. Quantitative digital subtraction radiography for the determination of small changes in bone thickness. Oral Surg Oral Med Oral Pathol Oral Radiol Endod. 1998; 85:462-72.
9. Bagchi P, Joshi N. Role of radiographic evaluation in treatment planning for dental implants: A review. J Dent Allied Sci 2012;1:21-5.
10. Frederiksen NL. Diagnostic imaging in dental implantology. Oral Surg Oral Med Oral Pathol Oral Radiol Endod 1995;80:540-54.
11. Tyndall DA, Brooks SL. Selection criteria for dental implant site imaging: A position paper of the American Academy of Oral and Maxillofacial radiology. Oral Surg Oral Med Oral Pathol Oral Radiol Endod 2000;89:630

12. Jayadevappa BS, Kodhandarama GS, Santosh SV. Imaging of dental implants .J *Oral Health* Res 2010;Vol 1(2).
13. Garg K. Dental Implant Imaging. Dent Implantol Update 2007;18(6).
14. Berger C, Duda M, Fleiner J. Three Dimentional Imaging In Dental Implantology. Eur J Oral Implantol 2009.
15. Miles DA. The future of dental and maxillofacial imaging. Dent Clin North Am 2008;52: 917-28.
16. Misch CE. Density of bone: Effect on treatment plans, surgical approach, healing, and progressive boen loading. Int J Oral Implantol 1990;6:23-31.
17. Sonick M, Abrahams J, Faiella RA. A comparison of the accuracy of periapical, panoramic, and computerized tomographic radiographs in locating the mandibular canal. Int J Oral Maxillofac Implants 1994; 9: 455-60.
18. Adell R, Lekholm U, Rockler B, Brånemark PI. A 15-year study of osseointegrated implants in the treatment of the edentulous jaw. Int J Oral Surg 1981;10: 387-416.
19. Engelman MJ, Sorensen JA, Moy P. Optimum placement of osseointegrated implants. J Prosthet Dent 1988;59:467-73.
20. Monsour PA, Dudhia R. Implant radiography and radiology. Aust Dent J 2008; 53 Suppl 1:S11-25.
21. Silverstein LH, Melkonian RW, Kurtzman D, Garnick JJ, Lefkove MD. Linear tomography in conjunction with pantomography in the assessment of dental implant recipient sites. J Oral Implantol 1994;20:111-7.
22. Meijer HJ, Steen WH, Bosman F. Standardized radiographs of the alveolar crest around implants in the mandible. J Prosthet Dent 1992;68: 318–321.
23. Chan HL, Misch K., Wang HL. Dental Imaging in Implant Treatment Planning. Implant Dent 2010 ;19:288-298.
24. Formoso N, Rilo B, Mora MJ, Martınez-Silva I,Santana U. A paralleling technique modification to determine the bone crest

level around dental implants. Dentomaxillofacial Radiol 2011 40, 385–389.

25. Lofthag-Hansen S, Lindh C, Petersson A. Radiographic assessment of the marginal bone level after implant treatment : a comparison of periapical and Scanora detailed narrow beam radiography. Dentomaxillofacial Radiol 2003;32:97-103.
26. Anil S,Al-Ghamadi H. A Method of Gauging Dental Radiographs during Treatment Planning for Dental Implants.J Contemp Dent Pract 2007 ;8(6) :082-088.
27. Kircos LT, Misch CE. Diagnostic imaging and techniques. In: Carl E. Misch. Dental Implant Prosthetics. Elsevier Mosby 2005:53-70.
28. Jameel N, Ibrahim O. Use of Longitudinal Topographic Occlusal Projection to measure the Alveolar Bone Thickness in the Posterior Implant Sites (Pre-Clinical Study).IJERSTE 2014; 3 (3): 1-7.
29. DulaE,MiniR,VanderPF,BuserD.Theradiographic assessment of implant patients: decision-making criteria. IntJOralMaxillofaclImpl 2001;16:8O–89.
30. Lindh C, Obrant K, Petersson A. Maxillary bone mineral density and its relationship to the bone mineral density of the lumbar spine and hip. Oral Surg Oral Med Oral Pathol Oral Radiol Endod, 2004;98:102-109.
31. Bolin A, Eliasson S, von Beetzen M, Jansson L. Radiographic evaluation of mandibular posterior implant sites: Correlation between panoramic and tomographic determinations. Clin Oral Implants Res 1996;7:354-9.
32. Bou Serhal C, Jacobs R, Persoons M, Hermans R, van SteenbergheD.Theaccuracyofspiraltomographytoassess bone quantity for the preoperative planning of implants in the posterior maxilla. Clin Oral Implants Res 2000; 11: 242–247.
33. White SC, Heslop EW, Hollender LG. American Academy of Oral and Maxillofacial Radiology, ad hoc Committee on Parameters of Care. Parameters of radiologic care: an official

report of the American Academy of Oral and Maxillofacial Radiology. Oral Surg Oral Med Oral Pathol Oral Radiol Endod. 2001;91:498-511.

34. Dharmar S. Locating the Mandibular Canal in Panoramic Radiographs. Int J Oral Maxillofac Implants 1997;12:113–117.
35. Vazquez L, Al Din Y, Belser U, Combescure C, Bernard J. Reliability of the vertical magnification factor on panoramic radiographs: clinical implications for posterior mandibular implants. Clin. Oral Impl. Res. 2011; 22: 1420–1425.
36. Gijbels F, Jacobs R, Bogaerts R, Debaveye D, Verlinden S, Sanderink G. Dosimetry of digital panoramic imaging. Part I: patient exposure. 2005; 34: 145–149.
37. Kim Y, Park J, Kim S, Kim J. Magnification rate of digital panoramic radiographs and its effectiveness for pre-operative assessment of dental implants. Dentomaxillofacial Radiol 2011; 40 :76–83.
38. Vazquez L, Nizamaldin Y, Combescure C, Nedir R, Bischof M, Dohan Ehrenfest D, etal. Accuracy of vertical height measurements on direct digital panoramic radiographs using posterior mandibular implants andmetal balls as reference objects. Dentomaxillofacial Radiol 2013; 42: 20110429.
39. Fortin T, Camby E, Alik M, Isidori M, Bouchet H. Panoramic Images versus Three-Dimensional Planning Software for Oral Implant Planning in Atrophied Posterior Maxillary: A Clinical Radiological Study. Clin Implant Dent Relat Res2013;15(2):198-204.
40. Penarrocha M, Palomar M, Sanchis M, Guarinos J, Balaguer J. Radiologic Study of Marginal Bone Loss Around 108 Dental Implants and Its Relationship to Smoking, Implant Location, and Morphology. Int J Oral Maxillofac Implants 2004;19:861–867.
41. Takeshita WM, Vessoni Iwaki L1, Da Silva M, Tonin R. Evaluation of diagnostic accuracy of conventional and digital periapical radiography, panoramic radiography, and

cone-beam computed tomography in the assessment of alveolar bone loss. Contemp Clin Dent.2014 ;5(3):318-323.

42. Strid KG, Branemark PI, Zarb G, Albrektsson T. Tissue-integrated prostheses: osseointegration in dentistry. *Quintessence Int* 1985: 187-98.
43. Fredholm U, Bolin A, Andersson L. Preimplant radiographic assessment of available maxillary bone support. Comparison of tomographic and panoramic technique. Swed Dent J 1993;17:103-9.
44. Shetty V, Benson BW. Oral radiology—principles and interpretation. In: White SC, Pharoah MJ 4th ed. St. Louis, Mosby 1999: 622-35.
45. Beltrao GC, de Abreu AT, Beltra RG, Finco NF. Lateral cephalometric radiograph for the planning of maxillary implant reconstruction. Dentomaxillofacial Radiol 2007; 36 :45–50.
46. Simon SS, Kumari R, Charllu A, Ramachandran S. A Cephalometric Technique to Aid in the Positioning of a Dental Implant. Journal of Scientific Dentistry 2013; 3(1):20-24.
47. Jacobs R, van Steenberghe D. Radiograpkic planningand assessment of endosseous oral implants, 1st edn. Berlin: Springer-Verlag,l998.
48. Schwarz MS, Rothman SL, Chafetz N, Stauts B. Preoperative diagnostic radiology for the tissue-integrated prosthesis. *Quintessence Int*1990:68-79.
49. Langland OE, Langlais RP, Mc David WD, Delbalso AM, editors. Panoramic radiology. 2nd ed. Philadelphia, Lea & Febiger; 1989.
50. Grondahl HG, Grondahl K, Webber RL. A digital subtraction technique for dental radiography. Oral Surg Oral Med Oral Pathol 1983; 5: 6-102.
51. Reddy MS, Wang IC. Radiographic determinants of implant performance. Adv Dent Res 1999; 13:136-45.

52. Vannier MW. Subtraction radiography. J Periodontol 1996; 67:949-50.
53. White SC, Pharoah MJ. Oral radiology principles and interpretation 5th edition, St. Louis, Mosby; 2004, P: 225-45.
54. Jung Y, Han C, Lee K. A 1-Year Radiographic Evaluation of Marginal Bone Around Dental Implants. Int J Oral Maxillofac Implants 1996;11:811–818.
55. Kwon J, Kim Y, Kim C. Assessing changes of peri-implant bone using digital subtraction radiography. J Korean Acad Prosthodont 2001; 39 (3):273-281.
56. Carneiro LS, da Cunha HA, Leles CR and Mendonc EF. Digital subtraction radiography evaluation of longitudinal bone density changes around immediate loading implants: a pilot study. 2012;41:241–247.
57. Bittar-Cortez J, Passeri L, Boscolo F, Haiter-Neto F. Comparison of hard tissue density changes around implants assessed in digitized conventional radiographs and subtraction images. Clin. Oral Impl. Res. 2006; 17 :560–564.
58. Bittar-Cortez J, Passeri L, de Almeida S, Haiter-Neto F. Comparison of peri-implant bone level assessment in digitized conventional radiographs and digital subtraction images. Dentomaxillofacial Radiol 2006; 35: 258–262.
59. Mehdizadeh M, Shirazi M, Farahbod F, Gholamrezaei. K. Comparative evaluation of peri-implant bone height in digital conventional radiographs and digital subtraction images. J Dent Implant2014 ;4 (1):11-15.
60. Brent Dove S, McDavid WD, Hamilton KE. Analysis of sensitivity and specificity of a new digital subtraction system. Oral Surg Oral Med Oral Pathol Oral Radiol Endod 2000; 89:771-6.
61. Wengraf A. Radiologically occult bone cavities: An experimental study and review. Br. Dent. J.1964; 117:532-6.

62. Sanz M, Newman MG. Advanced Diagnostic Techniques. In: Newman MG, Takei HH, and Carranza FA. Clinical periodontology.9th ed 2002 .p.487-502.
63. Masood F, Katz JO. Comparison of panoramic radiography and panoramic digital subtraction radiography in the detection of simulated osteophytic lesions of the mandibular condyle. Oral Surg Oral Med Oral Pathol Oral Radiol Endod, 2002; 93:626-31.
64. Sun HX, Ohki M, Yamada N. Quantitative evaluation of bone repaire of periapical lesions using digital subtraction radiography. Oral Radiol. 1991; 7:25-46.
65. Brooks SL. Maxillofacial Imaging. In Greenberg MS, Glick M. Burket"s oral medicine diagnosis and treatment. 10 ed,Ontario: BC Decker;2003.p.35-49.
66. Fidler A, Liker B. Influence of developer exhaustion on accuracy of quantitative digital subtraction radiography. Oral Surg Oral Med Oral Pathol Oral Radiol Endod 2000; 90: 233-9.
67. Berberi, A, Le Breton, G, Mani J, Woimant H. and Nasseh I. Lingual parasthesia following surgical placement of implants: report of a case. Int J Oral Maxillofac Implants 1993;8: 580–582.
68. Ellies, LG and Hawker PB. The prevalence of altered sensation associated with implant surgery. Int J Oral Maxillofac Implants 1993; 8:674–679.
69. Ten Bruggenkate CM, Krekeler G, Kraajenhagen HA, Foitzik C and Oosterbeek HS. Haemorrhage of the floor of the mouth resulting from lingual perforation during implant placement: a clinical report. Int J Oral Maxillofac Implants1993;8:329–334.
70. Regev E, Smith RA, Perrot DH and Pogrel MA. Maxillary sinus complications related to endosseous implants. Int J Oral Maxillofac Implants 1995; 10: 451–461.
71. Bloch F, Hansen W and Packard M. Nuclear induction. Physical Review 1946;69: 127.

72. Purcell EM, Torrey HC and Pound RV. Resonance absorption by nuclear magnetic moments in a solid. Physical Review 1946; 69: 37–38.
73. Damadian R. Tumor detection by nuclear magnetic resonance. Science 1971;171: 1151–1153.
74. Lauterbur PC. Image formation by induced local interactions: examples employing nuclear magnetic resonance. Nature 1973; 242: 190–191.
75. Edelstein WA, Hutchison JMS, Johnson G. & Redpath TW. Spin warp NMR imaging and applications to whole body imaging. Physics in Medicine and Biology 1980; 25: 751–766.
76. Hutchison JMS, Edelstein, WA, Johnson G. A whole body NMR imaging machine. Journal of Physics 1980; 13: 947–955.
77. Hawkes RC, Holland GN, Moore WS and Worthington BS. Nuclear magnetic resonance (NMR) tomography of the brain: a preliminary clinical assessment with demonstration of pathology. J Comput Assist Tomogr. 1980; 4: 577–586.
78. Young IR, Burl M, Clark GJ, Hall AS, Pasmore T and Collins AG. Magnetic resonance properties of hydrogen: imaging of the posterior fossa. Am J Roentgenol 1981;137: 895–901.
79. Katzberg RW. Temperomandibular joint imaging. Radiology 1989;170: 297–307.
80. Wortham DG, Teresi LM, Lufkin RB, Hanafee WN and Ward PH. Magnetic resonance imaging of the facial nerve. Otolaryngol Head Neck Surg.1989;101: 295–301.
81. Wong, W. (1996) Lower face and salivary glands. In: Edelman, R.R., Hesselink, J.R. & Zlatkin, M.B., eds. Clinical Magnetic Resonance Imaging, 2nd edn, 1996; 1:1110–1132.
82. Stark DD, Bradley WG. Magnetic Resonance Imaging.1999 St. Louis: C.V. Mosby.
83. McIsaac HK, Thordarson DS, Shafran R, Rachman S and Poole G. Claustrophobia and the magnetic resonance imaging procedure. J. Behav. Med. 1998;21: 255–268.

84. Jolesz F, Nabavi A and Kikinis R. Integration of interventional MRI with computer assisted surgery. J Magn Reson A. 2001;13: 69–77
85. Parkkola RK, Mattila KT, Ekfors TO, Komu MES, Vaara T and Aro HT. MR-guided core biopsies of soft tissue tumours on an open 0.23 T Imager. Acta Radiologica 2001;42: 302–305.
86. Spouse E and Gedroyc WM. MRI of the claustrophobic patient: interventionally configured magnets. Br J Radiol 2000;73: 146–151.
87. Lockhart PB, Kim S and Lund NL. Magnetic resonance imaging of human teeth.J Endod 1992;18: 237–244.
88. Baumann MA and Doll GM. Spatial reproduction of the root canal system by magnetic resonance microscopy. J Endod1997; 23: 49–51.
89. Aguiar M, Marques A, Carvalho A, Cavalcanti M. Accuracy of magnetic resonance imaging compared with computed tomography for implant planning. Clin. Oral Impl. Res. 2008 ;19: 362–365.
90. Gray C, Redpath T, Smith F. Low-field magnetic resonance imaging for implant dentistry. Contemp Clin Dent. 1998;27:225 - 229.
91. Gray C,Redpath T,Bainton R, Smith F. Magnetic resonance imaging assessment of a sinus lift operation using reoxidised cellulose (Surgicel) as graft material. Clin. Oral Impl. Res. 2001 ;12:526–530.
92. Pompa V, Galasso S, Cassetta M, Pompa G, Angelis F, Carlo S. A comparative study of Magnetic Resonance (MR) and Computed Tomography (CT) in the pre-implant evaluation. Annali di Stomatologia 2010; I (3-4): 33-38.
93. Imamura H, Sato H, Matsuura T, Ishikawa M, Zeze R. A Comparative Study of Computed Tomography and Magnetic Resonance Imaging for the Detection of Mandibular Canals

and Cross-Sectional Areas in Diagnosis prior to Dental Implant Treatment. Clin Implant Dent Relat Res 2004;6 (2):75-81.

94. Lindh C, Petersson R. Radiologic examination for location of the mandibular canal: a comparison between panoramic radiography and conventional tomography. Int J Oral Maxillofac Implants 1989; 4: S49–S53.
95. Klemetti E. Edentulous jaws and skeletal mineral status (Thesis). Euopio University Publications B, Dental Sciences 1993; 3:1-100.
96. Bou Serhal C, van Steenberghe D, Bosmans H, Sanderink GCH, Quirynen M, Jacobs R. Organ radiation dose assessment for conventional spiral tomography: a human cadaver study. Clin Oral Implants Res 2001; 12:85–9O.
97. Frederiksen NL. Advanced Imaging, In: Oral Radiology Principles and Interpretation,S.C. White & M. J. Pharoah, 2009: 207-224.
98. Jacobs R, Adriansens A, Naert I, Quirynen M, Hermans R, Steenberghe D. Predictability of reformatted computed tomography for pre-operative planning of endosseous implants. Dentomaxillofacial Radiol 1999; 28: 37 -41.
99. Ekestubbe A, Grondahl HG, Molander B. Quality of digital pre-implant tomography: comparison of film–screen images with storage phosphor images at normal. Dentomaxillofacial Radiol 2003; 32: 322–326.
100. Mraiwa N, Jacobs R, Cleynenbreuge J, Sanderink G, Schutyser F, Suetens P, Steenberghe D and Quirynen M. The nasopalatine canal revisited using 2D and 3D CT imaging. Dentomaxillofacial Radiol 2004; 33: 396–402.
101. Mathew A, Shenai P, Chatra L, Rao P, Prabhu R. Computed Tomographic Assessment of Lingual Vascular Channels in the Mandible – An Imaging Study. South East Asian J Clin Res 2015;1(1):11-15.
102. Dantas JA, Filho AM, Campos PSF. Computed tomography for dental implants: the influence of the gantry

angle and mandibular positioning on the bone height and width. Dentomaxillofacial Radiol 2005; 34: 9–15.

103. Ersoy A, Turkyilmaz I, Ozan O, McGlumphy EA.Reliability of Implant Placement With Stereolithographic Surgical Guides Generated From Computed Tomography: Clinical Data From 94 Implants. J Periodontol 2008;79:1339-1345.

104. Cuijpers V, Jaroszewicz J, Anil S, Aldosari A, Walboomers X, Jansen J. Resolution, sensitivity, and in vivo application of high-resolution computed tomography for titanium-coated polymethyl methacrylate (PMMA) dental implants. Clin. Oral Impl. Res. 2013 :1–7.

105. Schwarz MS, Rothman SL, Rhodes ML, Chafetz N. Computed tomography: part I. Preoperative assessment of the mandible for endosseous implant surgery. Int J Oral Maxillofac Implants 1987;2:137-41.

106. Klinge B, Petersson A, Maly P. Location of the mandibular canal: comparison of macroscopic findings, conventional radiography, and computed tomography. Int J Oral Maxillofac Implants 1989;4:327-32.

107. Littner MM, Kaffe I, Arensburg B, Calderon S, Levin T. Radiographic features of anterior buccal mandibular depression in modern human cadavers. Dentomaxillofac Radiol 1995;24:46-9.

108. Andersson JE, Svartz K. CT-scanning in the preoperative planning of osseointegrated implants in the maxilla. Int J Oral Maxillofac Surg 1988;17:33-5.

109. Arai Y, Tammisalo, E., Iwai, K.. Development of a compact computed tomographic apparatus for dental use. Dentomaxillofac Radiol 1999;28, 245-8.

110. Naitoh M, Hirukawa A, Katsumata A, Ariji E. Evaluation of voxel values in mandibular cancellous bone: Relationship between cone-beam computed tomography and multislice

helical computed tomography. Clin Oral Implants Res 2009; 20: 503-6.

111. Naitoh M, Hirukawa A, Katsumata A, Ariji E. Prospective study to estimate mandibular cancellous bone density using large-volume cone-beam computed tomography. Clin Oral Implants Res 2010; 21: 1309-13.

112. Mah P, Reeves TE, McDavid WD. Deriving Hounsfield units using grey levels in cone-beam computed tomography. Dentomaxillofac Radiol 2010; 39:323-35.

113. Katsumata A, Hirukawa, A, Okumura S, Naitoh M, Fujishita M, Ariji E, et al. Effects of image artifacts on gray-value density in limited-volume-cone-beam Computerized tomography. Oral Surg Oral Med Oral Pathol Oral Radiol Endod 2007;104: 829-36.

114. Ganz S. Computer-aided Design/Computer-aided Manufacturing Applications Using CT and Cone Beam CT Scanning Technology. Dent Clin N Am 2008; 52: 777-808.

115. Isoda K, Ayukawa Y, Tsukiyama Y, Sogo M, Matsushita Y, Koyano K. Relationship between the bone density estimated by cone-beam computed tomography and the primary stability of dental implants. Clin. Oral Impl. Res. 2012; 23: 832–83.

116. Parsa A,Ibrahim N,Hassan B, van der Stelt P,Wismeijer D. Bone quality evaluation at dental implant site using multislice CT, micro-CT, and cone beam CT. Clin. Oral Impl. Res. 2013 : 1–7.

117. Shiratori NL, Marotti J,Yamanouchi J, Chilvarquer I, Contin I, Tortamano-Neto P. Measurement of buccal bone volume of dental implants by means of cone-beam computed tomography. Clin. Oral Impl. Res. 2012; 23: 797–804.

118. Slagter KW, Raghoebar GM, Vissink A, Meijer H . Inter- and intraobserver reproducibility of buccal bone measurements at dental implants with cone beam computed

tomography in the esthetic region. *Int J* Oral Maxillofac *Implants* 2015; 1:8.

119. Ibrahim N, Parsa A,Hassan B, Stelt P,Aartman I, Wismeijer D. Accuracy of trabecular bone microstructural measurement at planned dental implant sites using cone-beam CT datasets. Clin. Oral Impl. Res. 2013 :1–5.

120. Fienitz T, Schwarz F, Ritter L, Dreiseidler T, Becker J, Rothamel D. Accuracy of cone beam computed tomography in assessing peri-implant bone defect regeneration: a histologically controlled study in dogs. Clin. Oral Impl. Res. 2012; 23: 882–887.

121. Kamburoglu K, Murat S, Kılıç C, Yuksel S, Avsever, H, Farman A, Scarfe WC. Accuracy of CBCT images in the assessment of buccal marginal alveolar peri-implant defects: effect of field of view. Dentomaxillofac Radiol 2014; 43: 20130332.

122. Corpas L, Jacobs R Quirynen M, Huang Y, Naert I. Duyck J. Peri-implant bone tissue assessment by comparing the outcome of intra-oral radiograph and cone beam computed tomography analyses to the histological standard. Clin. Oral Impl. Res. 2011; 22: 492–499.

123. Zhang W, Skrypczak A, Weltman R. Anterior maxilla alveolar ridge dimension and morphology measurement by cone beam computerized tomography (CBCT) for immediate implant treatment planning. BMC Oral Health 2015;15:65.

124. Janner S,Caversaccio M, Dubach P,Sendi P,Buser D,Bornstein MM. Characteristics and dimensions of the Schneiderian membrane: a radiographic analysis using cone beam computed tomography in patients referred for dental implant surgery in the posterior maxilla. Clin. Oral Impl. Res. 2011 ; 22:1446–1453.

125. Lana JP, Rodrigues PM, Carvalho, Machado Alencar de PE, Souza, Manzi FR, Rebello MC, Horta. Anatomic variations

and lesions of the maxillary sinus detected in cone beam computed tomography for dental implants. Clin. Oral Imp. Res. 2012 ; 22: 1398–1403.

126. Fornell J,Johansson L,Bolin A, Isaksson S, Sennerby L. Flapless, CBCT-guided osteotome sinus floor elevation with simultaneous implant installation. I: radiographic examination and surgical technique. A prospective 1-year follow-up. Clin. Oral Impl. Res. 2012; 23: 28–34.

127. Apostolakis D, Brown JE. The anterior loop of the inferior alveolar nerve: prevalence, measurement of its length and a recommendation for interforaminal implant installation based on cone beam CT imaging. Clin. Oral Impl. Res. 2012 ; 23: 1022–1030

128. Correa LR, Spin-Neto R, Stavropoulos A, Schropp L, Dias da HE, Silveira,et al. Planning of dental implant size with digital panoramic radiographs, CBCT-generated panoramic images,and CBCT cross-sectional images. Clin. Oral Impl. Res. 2013 : 1–6.

129. Suomalainen A, Vehmas T, Kortesniemi M, Robinson S, Peltola J. Accuracy of linear measurements using dental cone beam and conventional multislice computed tomography. Dentomaxillofac Radiol 2008 ;37:10–17.

130. Ken Yanagisawa, Craig D, Eugenia M, James J. Dentascan imaging of the mandible and maxilla. Head and Neck 2006;15(1):1-7.

131. Azari A, Nikzad S. Computerassisted implantology: historical background and potential outcomes - a review. Int J Med Robot 2008;4(2):95-104.

132. Jaju P,Suvarna P, Subramaniam A, Jaju S. Pre-evaluation of implant sites by Dentascans. J Dent Implant 2011 ;1 (2):64-74.

133. Klemetti E, Vainio P. Effect of maxillary edentulousness on mandibular residual ridges. Eur J Oral Sci. 1994;102(5):309-12.

134. Karl Dula, Roberto M, Jorg TL, Stelt PF, Schneeberger P, Clemens G, et al. Hypothetical mortality risk associated with spiral tomography of the maxilla and mandible prior to endosseous implant treatment. Eur J Oral Sci. 1997;105(2):123-29.

135. Chidiac JJ, Shofer FS, Al-Kutoubi A, Laster LL, Ghafari J. Comparison of CT scanograms and cephalometric radiographs in craniofacial imaging. Orthod Craniofac Res. 2002;5(2):104-13.

136. Tammisalo, E., Hallikainen, D., Kanerva, H., & Tammisalo, T. Comprehensive oral X-ray diagnosis: Scanora multimodal radiography. A preliminary description. Dentomaxillofac Radiol 1992; 21(1):9-15.

137. Gröndahl K, Ekestubbe A, Grondahl HG, Johnsson T. Reliability of hypocycloidal tomography for the evaluation of the distance from the alveolar crest to the mandibular canal. Dentomaxillofac Radiol 1991;20(4):200-4.

138. Cavalcanti MG, Vannier MW. Quantitative analysis of spiral computed tomography for craniofacial clinical applications. Dentomaxillofac Radiol 1998;27(6):344-50.

139. Diniz AF, Mendonça EF, Leles CR, Guilherme AS, Cavalcante MP, Silva MA. Changes in the pre-surgical treatment planning using conventional spiral tomography. Clin Oral Implants Res 2008;19(3):249-53.

140. Shahbazian M, Xue D, Hu Y, van Cleynenbreugel J, Jacobs R. Spiral computed tomography based maxillary sinus imaging in relation to tooth loss, implant placement and potential grafting procedure. J oral & maxillofac Res 2010;1(1):e7.

141. Chen LK, Su CT, Tsai YF, Chen HY, Lu CL, Lin CS, et al. Spiral Dental CT: Use in Evaluating Dental Implantation.2001;26(5):209-14.

142. Kassebaum DK, Stoller NE, McDavid WD, Goshorn B, Ahrens CR. Absorbed dose determination for tomographic implant site assessment techniques. Oral Surg. Oral Med. Oral Pathol. 1992;73(4):502-9.

143. Eckerdal O, Kvint S. "Presurgical planning for osseointegrated implants in the maxilla: a tomographic evaluation of available alveolar bone and morphological relations in the maxilla." Int J *Oral* Maxillofac Surg 1986; 722-726.

144. Rockenbach M, Sampaio M, Costa L, Costa N. Evaluation of Mandibular Implant Sites: Correlation between Panoramic and Linear Tomography. Braz Dent J 2003; 14(3): 209-213.

145. Todd A, Gher M, Quintero G, Richardsorf A. Interpretation of Linear and Computed Tomograms in the Assessment of Implant Recipient Sites. J Periodontol 1993;64: 1243-1249.

146. Schwarz MS, Rothman SL, Chafetz N, Rhodes M. Computed tomography in dental implantation surgery. Dent Clin North Am 1989;33:555-97.

147. Gröndahl K, Ekestubbe A, Gröndahl HG, Johnsson T. Reliability of hypocycloidal tomography for the evaluation of the distance from the alveolar crest to the mandibular canal. Dentomaxillofac Radiol 1991;20:200-4.

148. Peltola JS, Mattila M. Cross-sectional tomograms obtained with four panoramic radiographic units in the assessment of implant site Measurements. Dentomaxillofac Radiol 2004 ;33: 295–300.

149. Bousquet F, Bousquet P, L Vazquez. Transtomography for implant placement guidance in non-invasive surgical procedures. Dentomaxillofac Radiol 2007; 36 :229–233.

150. Welander U, Li G, Mc David WD, Tronje G. Transtomography : a new tomographic scanning technique . Dentomaxillofacial Radiol 2004; 33:188-195.

151. Dreiseidler T, Mischkowski RA, Neugebauer J, Ritter L, Zöller JE. Comparison of cone-beam imaging with

orthopantomography and computerized tomography for assessment in presurgical implant dentistry. Int J Oral Maxillofac Implants 2009;24:216-25.

152. Chau AC, Fung K. Comparison of radiation dose for implant imaging using conventional spiral tomography, computed tomography, and cone-beam computed tomography. Oral Surg Oral Med Oral Pathol Oral Radiol Endod 2009;107:559-65.

153. Moussa R, Awadalla M, Marei M, Nassef T. A Computerized Tomographic Data Analysis System to Evaluate the Dental Implant Surface Roughness. Procedia Computer Science 2015 ; 61:472 – 477.

154. Geng W, Liu C, Su Y, Li J, Zhou Y. Accuracy of different types of computer-aided design/ computer-aided manufacturing surgical guides for dental implant placement.Int J Clin Exp Med 2015;8(6):8442-8449.

155. Moustafa R, Nassef T, Alkhodary M, Marei M, Awadalla M.A New Interactive 3-D Numerical Model of the Human Mandible for Peri-Implant Analysis in-Vivo Compared With Cone Beam Computed Tomography 3-D Quality. J Biomed Eng; 2012; 2(1): 9-16.

156. Yatzkair G, Cheng A, Brodie S, Raviv E, Boyan B, Schwartz Z. Accuracy of computer-guided implantation in a human cadaver model. Clin. Oral Impl. Res. 2015; 26:1143–1149.

157. Verstreken K, Van Cleynenbreugel J, Marchal G, Naert I, Suetens P, van Steenberghe D. Computer-assisted planning of oral implant surgery: a three-dimensional approach. Int J Oral Maxillofac Implants 1996;11:806-10.

158. Lambrecht JT, Hammer B, Jacob AL, et al. Individual model fabrication in maxillofacial radiology. Dentomaxillofac Radiol 1995;24:147-54.

159. Sudbrink SD. Computer-guided implant placement with immediate provisionalization: a case report. J Oral Maxillofac Surg 2005;63:771-4.

160. Petrikowski CG et al. Presurgical radiographic assessment for implants. J Prosthet Dent 1989;61(1):59-64.

161. Campelo LD, Camara JR. Flapless implant surgery: a 10-year clinical retrospective analysis. Int J Oral Maxillofac Implants. 2002;17:271–276.

162. Rocci A, Martignoni M, Gottlow J. Immediate loading in the maxilla using flapless surgery, implants placed in predetermined positions, and prefabricated provisional restorations: a retrospective 3-year clinical study. Clin Implant Dent Relat Res. 2003;5(Suppl.):29–36.

163. Borrow JW, Smith JP. Stent marker materials for computerized tomograph-assisted implant planning. Int J Periodontics Restorative Dent 1996; 16:60–67.

164. Cassetta M, Carlo S, Pranno N, Sorrentino V, Giorgio G,Pompa G. The use of stereolithographic surgical templates in oral implantology. Ann. Ital. Chir., 2013; 84(5).

165. Schropp L, Stavropoulos A, Gotfredsen E, Wenzel A. Calibration of radiographs by a reference metal ball affects preoperative selection of implant size. Clin Oral Invest 2009; 13:375–381.

166. Ozan O, Turkyilmaz I, Yilmaz B. A preliminary report of patients treated with early loaded implants using computerized tomography-guided surgical stents: flapless versus conventional flapped surgery. J Oral Rehabil 2007; 34:835–840.

167. Lal K, White GS, Morea DN, Wright RF. Use of stereolithographic templates for surgical and prosthodonticimplant planning and placement. Part I. The concept. J Prosthodont. 2006;15:51–58.

168. Gray CF, Redpath TW, Smith FW. Pre-surgical dental implant assessment by magnetic resonance imaging. J Oral Implantol 1996;22:147-53.

169. Zhao XZ, Hua XUW, Tang ZH, Wu MJ, Zhu, Chen S. Accuracy of Computer-Guided Implant Surgery by a CAD/CAM and Laser Scanning Technique.Chin J Dent Res 2014; 17(1).

170. Ruppin J, Popovic A, Strauss M, Spuntrup E, Steiner A, Stoll C. Evaluation of the accuracy of three different computer-aided surgery systems in dental implantology: optical tracking vs. stereolithographic splint systems. Clin. Oral Impl. Res. 2008 ;(19): 709–716.

171. Fortin T, Champleboux G,Bianchi S,Buatois H,Coudert J. Precision of transfer of preoperative planning for oral implants based on cone-beam CT-scan images through a robotic drilling machine:An in vitro study. Clin. Oral Impl. Res. 2002; 13: 651–656.

172. Wanschitz F, Birkfellner W, Figl M, Patruta S, Wagner A, Watzinger F, et al. Computer-enhanced stereoscopic vision in a head-mounted display for oral implant surgery. Clin. Oral Impl. Res. 2002;13: 610–616.

www.ingramcontent.com/pod-product-compliance
Ingram Content Group UK Ltd.
Pitfield, Milton Keynes, MK11 3LW, UK
UKHW041853190726
13854UKWH00002B/871

9 789354 461989